Medical Economics Company Inc.
Book Division
Oradell, New Jersey 07649

Edited by John T. Queenan, M.D.

A
CONTEMPORARY OB/GYN
BOOK
Managing Ob/Gyn EMERGENCIES

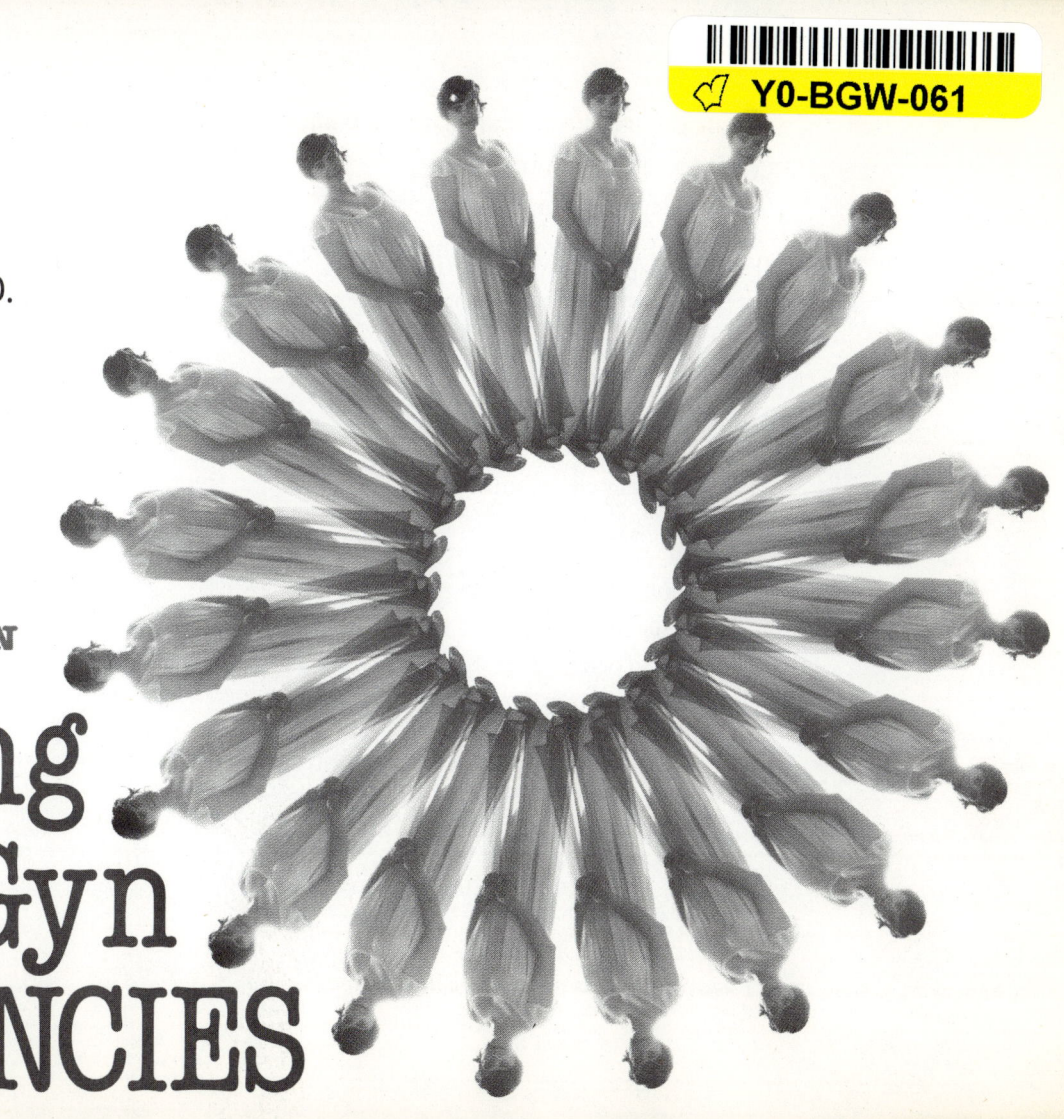

Library of Congress Cataloging in Publication Data

Main entry under title:

Managing ob/gyn emergencies.

  Text adapted from the special issue on emergencies of Contemporary ob/gyn, v. 18, July 1981.
   "A Contemporary ob/gyn book."
   Includes bibliographical references and index.
   1. Pregnancy, Complications of. 2. Labor, Complicated. 3. Gynecologic emergenices. I. Queenan, John T. II. Contemporary ob/gyn. III. Title: Managing obstetrics/gynecology emergencies. [DNLM: 1. Emergencies. 2. Genital diseases, Female—Therapy. 3. Pregnancy complications—Therapy. WQ 240 M267]
RG571.M27   618.3'025   81-16814
ISBN 0-87489-273-2   AACR2

Design by Elaine Kilcullen

Cover photograph by Doug Bates

ISBN 0-87489-273-2

Medical Economics Company Inc.
Oradell, New Jersey 07649

Printed in the United States of America

First Printing   January, 1982
Second Printing   September, 1982

Copyright © 1982 by Medical Economics Company Inc., Oradell, N.J. 07649. All rights reserved. None of the content of this publication may be reproduced, stored in a retrieval system, or transmitted in any form or by any means (electronic, mechanical, photocopying, recording, or otherwise) without the prior written permission of the publisher.

Contents

Contributors/Participants   vi

Preface: Knowledge, experience, and reflexes.
John T. Queenan, MD   ix

1. CPR for vasovagal syncope.
   J. Stephen Naulty, MD, and Gerard W. Ostheimer, MD   1

2. How to manage acute renal failure.
   Kenneth A. Fisher, MD   9

3. Anesthetic emergencies.
   Raymond R. Schultetus, MD, PhD   17

4. Responding to cardiorespiratory complications.
   Robert H. Hayashi, MD   27

5. Managing acute abdominal problems in pregnancy.
   Gail V. Anderson, MD, and Alan Ball, PA-C   37

6. How good is emergency training for ob/gyn residents? 49

7. Treatment priorities for the ob patient in shock.
Denis Cavanagh, MD, and Robert A. Knuppel, MD, MPH 55

8. Detecting and treating ectopic pregnancy.
Gregory C. Bolton, MD, and Fredric L. Cohen, MD 63

9. Surgery for ruptured pelvic abscesses?
F. Gary Cunningham, MD, and David L. Hemsell, MD 71

10. How to cope with hemorrhage.
Walter B. Jones, MD 79

11. Managing anovulatory bleeding medically.
Leon Speroff, MD 85

12. Fetal bradycardia: Watch or deliver?
Edward J. Quilligan, MD 91

13. Strategies for controlling eclampsia.
Frederick P. Zuspan, MD, and Kathryn J. Zuspan, MD 99

14. Ruptured uterus: Still a challenge.
Mary Jo O'Sullivan, MD 107

15. Fast action for the distressed newborn.
John W. Scanlon, MD 115

16. Postpartum endometritis.
    Philip B. Mead, MD   125

17. Problem-patient conference: Subarachnoid hemorrhage in pregnancy.
    Ralph M. Richart, MD, editor   133

    Index   149

Contributors/Participants

Gail V. Anderson, MD, Director of Emergency, LAC/USC Medical Center; Chairman and Professor, Department of Emergency Medicine, University of Southern California School of Medicine, Los Angeles

John L. Antunes, MD, Associate Professor of Neurological Surgery and assistant attending Neurological surgeon, Neurological Institute of New York, Columbia University College of Physicians and Surgeons

Hervy E. Averette, MD, Professor and Director, Division of Gynecologic Oncology, University of Miami School of Medicine, Miami, Florida

Alan Ball, PA-C, Emergency medicine physician's assistant resident, LAC/USC Medical Center, Los Angeles

Bruce A. Barron, MD, PhD, Associate Professor of Obstetrics and Gynecology, Columbia University College of Physicians and Surgeons, New York

Thomas J. Benedetti, MD, Assistant Professor of Obstetrics and Gynecology, University of Washington School of Medicine, Seattle

Gregory C. Bolton, MD, Assistant Professor of Obstetrics and Gynecology, University of Pennsylvania School of Medicine, Philadelphia

Denis Cavanagh, MD, Professor of Obstetrics and Gynecology and Director, Division of Gynecologic Oncology, University of South Florida College of Medicine, Tampa

Fredric L. Cohen, MD, Senior Resident, Department of Obstetrics and Gynecology, Pennsylvania Hospital, Philadelphia

Joseph Collea, MD, Director of Residency Training, Georgetown University School of Medicine, Washington, D.C.

F. Gary Cunningham, MD, Professor of Obstetrics and Gynecology, University of Texas Health Science Center, Dallas

S. Ender Dolen, MD, Assistant Professor of Obstetrics and Gynecology, Texas Tech University Health Science Center; Director of the Residency Program, Lubbock General Hospital, Lubbock

Mieczyslaw Finster, MD, Professor of Anesthesiology and Obstetrics and Gynecology; Director, Obstetrical Anesthesia Service, Presbyterian Hospital, Columbia University College of Physicians and Surgeons, New York

Kenneth A. Fisher, MD, Academic Director of Internal Medicine, University of Illinois at MacNeal Memorial Hospital, Berwyn

Robert H. Hayashi, MD, Associate Professor of Obstetrics and Gynecology, University of Texas Health Science Center, San Antonio

David L. Hemsell, MD, Assistant Professor of Obstetrics and Gynecology, University of Texas Health Science Center, Dallas

Walter B. Jones, MD, Associate Professor of Obstetrics and Gynecology, Cornell University Medical College; associate attending surgeon, Memorial Sloan-Kettering Cancer Center, New York

Robert A. Knuppel, MD, MPH, Associate Professor of Obstetrics and Gynecology and Director, Division of Maternal-Fetal Medicine, University of South Florida College of Medicine, Tampa

Philip B. Mead, MD, Professor and Director of Residency Training, Department of Obstetrics and Gynecology, University of Vermont College of Medicine, Burlington

J. Stephen Naulty, MD, Instructor of Anesthesia, Harvard Medical School, Boston

Gerard W. Ostheimer, MD, Assistant Professor of Anesthesia, Harvard Medical School; Associate Director of Obstetrical Anesthesia, Brigham and Women's Hospital, Boston

Mary Jo O'Sullivan, MD, Associate Professor and Director of Clinical Perinatology, University of Miami School of Medicine, Miami, Florida

Roy H. Petrie, MD, Associate Professor of Obstetrics and Gynecology, Columbia University College of Physicians and Surgeons; Section of Perinatal Obstetrics, Department of Obstetrics and Gynecology, Sloane Hospital for Women, New York

John T. Queenan, MD, Professor and Chairman, Department of Obstetrics and Gynecology, Georgetown University School of Medicine, Washington, D.C., and Editor-in-Chief, CONTEMPORARY OB/GYN

Edward J. Quilligan, MD, Professor of Obstetrics and Gynecology and head of the Division of Maternal-Fetal Medicine, University of California Irvine Medical Center, Orange

Ralph M. Richart, MD, Professor of Pathology, Division of Obstetric-Gynecologic Pathology and Cytology, Columbia-Presbyterian Medical Center, New York

John W. Scanlon, MD, Associate Professor of Pediatrics, Georgetown University School of Medicine; Director of Neonatology, Columbia Hospital for Women, Washington, D.C.

Raymond R. Schultetus, MD, PhD, Assistant Professor of Anesthesiology, University of Florida College of Medicine, Gainesville

Leon Speroff, MD, Professor and Chairman, Department of Obstetrics and Gynecology, University of Oregon School of Medicine, Portland

Raymond Vande Wiele, MD, Professor and Chairman, Department of Obstetrics and Gynecology, Columbia University College of Physicians and Surgeons, New York

Frederick P. Zuspan, MD, Professor and Chairman, Department of Obstetrics and Gynecology, Ohio State University, Columbus

Kathryn J. Zuspan, MD, resident, Department of Obstetrics and Gynecology, University of North Carolina Medical School, Chapel Hill

Preface: Knowledge, experience, and reflexes

Obstetrics and gynecology is a unique specialty. Its practice covers the full spectrum of care—medical, surgical, psychological. The emergencies we're called upon to handle occur over the entire area of practice. We must, therefore, have a broad background if we're to be prepared to handle the unexpected. And the emergencies, as we all know, commonly occur in the middle of the night. It's not unusual for an obstetrician-gynecologist to be the only physician immediately available in the hospital at night.

There are two types of emergencies in obstetrics and gynecology—the immediate and the imminent. Immediate emergencies allow no time for review. You must react fast. Seconds count! Success depends on your perspicacity, know-how, and reflexes. With luck, you can muster a team to assist you. The life-threatening immediate emergencies include anesthetic catastrophies, distress in neonates, thromboembolic phenomena, eclampsia, and amniotic fluid emboli.

The imminent emergencies may be equally life-threatening, but you have a little time to organize a plan. Here, minutes count! Success depends on your knowledge and skill, and whether you can get the best help available. The life-threatening imminent emergencies include acute abdominal complications, ruptured tubo-ovarian abscess, shock, and severe bleeding.

I'll never forget my first night as a medical intern at Bellevue Hospital in New York. I raced to the emergency room to see an 18-year-old man in severe diabetic acidosis and with overwhelming, bilateral, pneumococcal pneumonia. It was obvious that this patient was very close to death. Being a relatively alert person, I knew just what to do. I turned around and said, "Get a doctor!" Then I realized I *was* the doctor. It was a very unsettling feeling.

Being prepared for a wide range of emergencies is a major undertaking. We've all learned to manage each of the emergencies that arise in obstetrics and gynecology. But the key to reacting well is to stay current. Probably physicians are best prepared to meet emergencies during the last year of residency or the first year as an attending. Then, unless you make special efforts, your skills will suffer from disuse.

How to remain current—that's a major concern. One step is to take a course in cardiopulmonary resuscitation, or better yet, one in advanced CPR. Chapter 6 surveys the attitudes of experts from both large and small institutions on how to improve emergency training for ob/gyn residents. Others focus on the specifics of how to handle the immediate and the imminent crises that will continually test your skills and resources.

To have a broad enough base to handle all ob-gyn emergencies, you need to participate in continuing medical education on a regular basis. The purpose of this book, adapted from a special issue of *Contemporary Ob/Gyn*, is to contribute to the clinician's CME in emergencies. I hope it will be helpful in bringing you up to date in the management of obstetric and gynecologic crises.

What about the 18-year-old patient? He did very well. I initiated care and got additional help fast. But that night I realized there are some things doctors must be prepared to do by reflex.

John T. Queenan, MD

J. Stephen Naulty, MD
Gerard W. Ostheimer, MD

CPR for vasovagal syncope

This poorly defined but very real syndrome can be fatal. You can reduce the likelihood you'll encounter it, and its severity if you do, by taking a good history and using premedication judiciously. Patients who have an attack should be managed by basic principles of CPR.

Vasovagal syncope arrives without warning. Its duration is brief, and its effects unpredictable. Attempts to reproduce it in susceptible individuals have not succeeded.

Two conditions appear necessary. First, there must be actual or a threat of physical injury. The threat or injury is most likely to produce vasovagal syncope if it involves new experience or one the patient has been unable to manage in the past. Second, the injury must be one the patient is expected to face easily.[1] For example, most people would not faint at venipuncture, injection of a local anesthetic, or even the sight of a needle (Figure 1-1). However, these seemingly trivial procedures may overwhelm susceptible individuals. For this reason, the syndrome is more common in men than women. In our society, men are expected to withstand such insults more readily.

Pathophysiology

The attack appears to involve a biphasic response.[2,3] First, there must be a massive discharge from the sympathetic nervous system in response to the threat of physical injury. The pulse rate, blood pressure (systolic

Figure 1-1. A classic case

A 17-year old high school senior comes to her gynecologist's office for a therapeutic abortion. She tells the nurse she always faints at the sight of needles or when blood has been drawn from her. On the examining table, she appears agitated and tremulous. The procedure is started under paracervical block anesthesia. As the first dose of local anesthetic is given, the patient appears diaphoretic and pale. During the injection, she loses consciousness and has a grand mal seizure. Following the seizure, the patient is apneic, with no pulses palpable and pupils widely dilated. An ECG reveals asystole. Cardiopulmonary resuscitation is quickly instituted and within 35 minutes the patient regains consciousness. Fifteen minutes later, her recovery appears complete with no neurologic sequelae and she insists on going home. A week later, she undergoes an uneventful therapeutic abortion, under general anesthesia, in the hospital.

---

greater than diastolic), and cardiac output all increase. And there is a massive increase in systemic vascular resistance. The patient appears apprehensive and pale, but usually denies any stress. Then, the physical changes suddenly reverse—as though the organism gives up in the face of an overwhelming threat.

As Figure 1-2 shows, pulse, blood pressure, cardiac output, and systemic vascular resistance suddenly drop. At the same time, the capacitance of the venous system suddenly increases, which leads to circulatory failure. The patient feels weak and diaphoretic, has a sudden decrease in muscle strength, becomes lightheaded, complains of vertigo, and quickly loses consciousness as the systolic pressure declines below 80 torr. The syncopal episode may be accompanied by vomiting, seizures, and a bowel movement (Table 1-1). If the response is sufficiently severe, "sudden death" may occur. This sequence has been described in patients who suddenly die in the coronary care unit.[4]

This biphasic response has been related to the sudden activation of the fight-or-flight mechanism of the sympathetic nervous system, abruptly followed by the activation of the

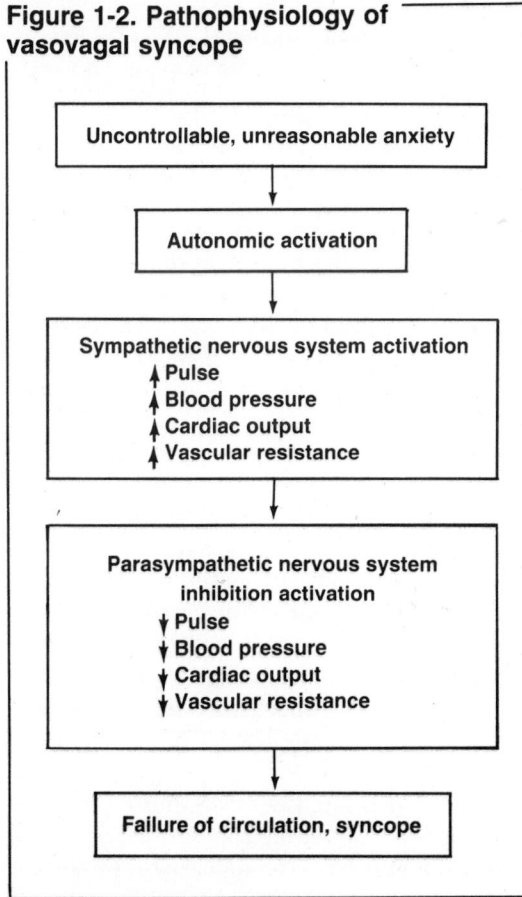

Figure 1-2. Pathophysiology of vasovagal syncope

vagal conservation-withdrawal system. Under normal circumstances, activation of the sympathetic nervous system inhibits the parasympathetic nervous system and vice versa.[1] Under conditions of conflicting stimulation, when the organism is faced with overwhelming terror at an apparently trivial stimulus, this reciprocal inhibition may begin to break down.[5]

If both systems are activated concurrently, a syncopal episode results. For instance, a terrified dog may bark and exhibit aggressive tendencies and simultaneously urinate, defecate, pant, salivate, move aimlessly, and even momentarily doze. The analogous hu-

Table 1-1. Symptoms of vasovagal syncope

Sympathetic activation	Parasympathetic activation
Trembling	Diminished muscle tone, weakness
Diaphoresis	
Pallor	Urination
Hyperventilation	Loss of bowel control
Piloerection	Loss of consciousness
	Bradycardia

man response, vasovagal syncope, may represent the organism's extreme reaction to overwhelming uncertainty about whether fighting or giving up is the best response to overwhelming stress.

The ABCs of managing a vasovagal attack

Despite uncertainty about its pathophysiology, the management of vasovagal syncope is fairly straightforward. The chief ingredients are the skills and equipment needed for cardiopulmonary resuscitation (CPR) (Table 1-2). The familiar ABCs of CPR provide an excellent framework for the management of vasovagal syncope.

Assessment. Place the patient supine, preferably with the head down. Check quickly for pulse, respiration, and level of consciousness. In basic CPR this means asking patients if they are all right, listening for respiration, and palpating a carotid pulse. If you've already attached an ECG monitor, consult the tracings, but don't take the time to attach one. In vasovagal syncope, you can expect an unconscious, apneic patient with a slow or nonpalpable or absent pulse.

Airway. After quick assessment, establish an airway. The American Heart Association (AHA) recommends the victim's head "be tilted backward as far as possible."[6] If this doesn't clear the airway, use the jaw-thrust maneuver. If she has vomited, remove the vomitus from the upper airway. Once these maneuvers are accomplished, quickly do a reassessment.

Breathing. If the patient does not rapidly begin to breathe spontaneously after you've established an airway, you must take the second

---

Table 1-2. ABCs of managing vasovagal syncope

Assess: Respiration, pulse, level of consciousness, and ECG (if possible).
Airway: Extend head, or use jaw-thrust maneuver.
Breathing: Begin mouth-to-mouth resuscitation, or artificial intermittent positive pressure breathing with oxygen.
Circulation: Perform external cardiac compression, 60 to 80 times per minute.
Drugs: Administer atropine (0.5 to 1.0 mg IV) or epinephrine (0.5 mg IV).
Electricity: Apply direct current defibrillation (200 to 400 joules).

step in CPR: Initiate breathing. How this is accomplished depends on the equipment available, but don't delay artificial respiration merely to obtain equipment.

The AHA recommends delivering four rapid breaths (mouth-to-mouth or by bag and mask) immediately following establishment of an airway. Follow this cycle by one breath every 5 seconds until spontaneous respirations resume. Palpate the carotid pulse again, and, if it's absent, go to the third step in CPR: Initiate circulation.[4]

Circulation. If the carotid pulse is absent, or even if there is a questionable pulse, you should use external cardiac compression to produce an artificial circulation. The AHA defines external cardiac compression as "the rhythmic application of pressure over the lower one half of the sternum, but not over the xyphoid process."[6] This maneuver should be performed 60 times a minute when two people are available, or 80 times a minute when only one is available. Always give external cardiac compression concomitantly with artificial ventilation. The techniques for doing this are well detailed in the AMA's *Standards for Cardiopulmonary Resuscitation*.[6] If after a few minutes of external compression there still is no cardiac activity, go to the fourth step in CPR: drug therapy.

Drugs. The usual cardiovascular event in vasovagal syncope is cardiac asystole or a profound bradycardia. Once you establish adequate circulation and ventilation, administer atropine IV, 0.5 to 1 mg. Repeat at 5-minute intervals until a pulse rate greater than 60 is established. Normally, the total dose of atropine should not exceed 2 mg. If atropine does not restore cardiac rhythm, further interventions will be necessary.

The interventions presuppose knowledge of the ECG and the ability to defibrillate the heart. Therefore, procedures likely to produce vasovagal syncope, such as the injection of local anesthetic or painful procedures, should be performed only when an ECG machine and a defibrillator are available. If the ECG reveals asystole and it is unresponsive to atropine, then inject IV 0.5 mg epinephrine to convert the asystole to ventricular fibrillation.

Electrical defibrillation. If a patient is found in ventricular fibrillation, or if epinephrine has converted asystole fibrillation, then perform direct current defibrillation using a delivered dose of 200 to 400 joules (W/second). If an ECG is unavailable and the patient has been unresponsive to atropine, then give a dose of epinephrine and make one unmonitored defibrillation attempt.

Differential diagnosis

Many conditions may mimic vasovagal syncope. The common ones include local anesthetic toxicity, profound hyperventilation, and myocardial infarction.

Local anesthetic toxicity. The accidental injection of a local anesthetic drug IV may produce symptoms like vasovagal syncope: agitation, tremulousness, and cardiorespiratory collapse with a seizure. What distinguishes the anesthetic reaction is that it occurs in the absence of a history of fainting and without the signs of anxiety and terror that usually precede a vasovagal attack. The management of the two conditions, however, is similar, applying the basic steps of CPR. The anesthetic problem is usually brief and self-limited. If she breathes sufficient oxygen and the pulse is maintained, the patient will quickly recover consciousness.

Hyperventilation. An extremely anxious patient may hyperventilate and lose consciousness as a result of intense cerebral vasoconstriction. This is usually a self-limited event. After this type of fainting, arterial CO_2 accumulates, vasoconstriction decreases, and the patient regains consciousness. Again, the management of hyperventilation syncope is the same as that of vasovagal syncope. Establish an airway and the patient will quickly begin breathing.

Myocardial infarction. A patient undergoing a stressful procedure, who has coronary artery disease, may develop a myocardial infarction during the procedure. Many of the same symptoms as vasovagal syncope may be produced, and, in fact, the myocardial infarction may result from the same mechanism that produces the vasovagal episode. The intense vasoconstriction and increased cardiac output stress initiates may increase the heart's oxygen requirements above what a compromised coronary circulation can provide. Myocardial ischemia and infarction may ensue, followed by vasomotor collapse, bradycardia, and profound hypotension. The patient's age, sex, and history may help you diagnose myocardial infarction.

CPR must be instituted and continued in either case, but recovery may take longer with a myocardial infarction. The patient who has had a heart attack will probably regain consciousness complaining of chest pain. If there is any doubt about whether the episode was vasovagal or myocardial, you should transfer the patient to a hospital for further evaluation and observation.

Guidelines to prevention

A patient who gives a history of fainting under stressful circumstances, or who appears more anxious than the nature of the procedure would warrant, may be considered susceptible to a vasovagal attack. Reviewing the entire procedure, giving reassurance, and encouraging questions may be helpful. An informative interview has been found most effective in reducing anxiety.[7] Premedication with tranquilizers or sedative drugs, in combination with atropine, may also help reduce the incidence or severity of attacks in susceptible individuals. Finally, when you prepare to do a potentially stressful procedure on a patient with a history of syncope, set up ECG monitoring before you begin.

REFERENCES
1. Engel GL: Psychologic stress, vasodepressor (vasovagal) syncope and sudden death. Ann Intern Med 89:403, 1978
2. Graham DT, Kabler JD, Lunsford L: Vasovagal fainting: A biphasic response. Psychosom Med 23:493, 1961
3. Tizes R: Cardiac arrest following routine venipuncture. JAMA 236:1846, 1976
4. Wolf S: Central autonomic influences on cardiac rate and rhythm. Mod Concepts Cardiovasc Dis 38:29, 1969
5. Gellhorn E: *Principles of Autonomic-Somatic Integrations.* Minneapolis: University of Minnesota Press, 1967
6. Standards for Cardiopulmonary Resuscitation (CPR) and Emergency Cardiac Care (EEC). JAMA 227:833, 1974
7. Egbert LD, Battit GE, Turndoff H, et al: The value of the pre-operative visit. JAMA 185:553, 1963

Kenneth A. Fisher, MD

How to manage acute renal failure

2

After identifying the initiating complication, monitor fluid overload, electrolyte or acid-base imbalance, and uremia. If artificial renal support is necessary, you'll have to choose between hemo- and peritoneal dialysis.

Any deterioration of renal function, with or without oliguria, poses a serious obstetric problem. Obstetrician and nephrologist must work closely together. The nephrologist is best equipped to deal with the metabolic aberrations caused by renal failure, while the obstetrician has the skills to treat the underlying systemic pathology. In most cases, the patient's survival depends on managing these problems successfully.

Contrary to what clinicians used to believe, pregnancy without further complications does not exacerbate pre-existing renal disease—even in systemic lupus erythematosus.[1] Increasing proteinuria, which is secondary to the physiologic increase in glomerular filtration rate, was in good part responsible for this misconception.[2] However, severe hypertension, especially if uncontrolled, can in itself cause a decrease in renal function. Also, the pregnant woman is susceptible to any of the renal diseases seen in the general population.[3] Still, most problems that are known to be associated with renal function in pregnant women are related to one of the various complications of pregnancy.

Diagnosing the specific syndrome

Two diseases associated with pregnancy can lead to renal failure, without additional obstetric complications. Preeclampsia-eclampsia, a systemic hypertensive disease of unknown etiology, is associated with a relatively specific renal lesion.[4] This disease can be complicated by acute renal failure, which is frequently the result of tubular necrosis (usually reversible). Occasionally, renal failure is caused by bilateral cortical necrosis. This often progresses to chronic renal failure. Preeclampsia is difficult to diagnose clinically, especially in the multipara. Nor is it easy to differentiate preeclampsia clinically from nephrosclerosis (hypertensive kidney) or other underlying renal disease.[5] These entities, when superimposed on preeclampsia, may have a higher incidence of acute renal failure.[6]

Postpartum renal failure, another pregnancy-specific syndrome, frequently results in kidney failure. This relatively rare syndrome may be associated with microangiopathic hemolytic anemia.[7] It usually does not resolve, thereby requiring dialysis or transplantation to maintain life. Two pathologic patterns have emerged. One resembles thrombotic microangiopathy;[7] the other is a nephrosclerotic picture much like scleroderma.[8] Whether these two lesions represent a different time course in the same disease or separate diseases is not yet known. Some authors, who do not consider postpartum renal failure a specific disease, have classified various lesions under this heading.[9] Experience with heparin therapy in these patients has been inconsistent, and if a subset of patients exists who would benefit from such therapy, they are yet to be defined.

Other pregnancy-associated entities can lead to acute renal failure as the result of the additional complications of coagulation defects, ischemia, or infection (Table 2-1). Abruptio placentae, prolonged intrauterine fetal death, and amniotic fluid embolism probably cause renal failure through alterations in coagulation. Infection, as a result of puerperal sepsis, pyelonephritis, chorioamnionitis, and septic abortion (early in pregnancy), may cause renal failure, with or without associated disseminated intravascular coagulation. Ischemic renal damage may accompany postpartum hemorrhage, placenta previa, and hyperemesis gravidarum. Renal failure associated with fatty liver and jaundice of pregnancy probably results from the same mechanism as any severe hepatic failure.

Table 2-1. Conditions associated with acute renal failure in pregnancy

Placenta previa
Abruptio placentae
Postpartum hemorrhage
Hyperemesis gravidarum
Preeclampsia-eclampsia
Abortion
    Septic
    Hemorrhage
    Toxins
Puerperal sepsis
Chorioamnionitis
Pyelonephritis
Disseminated intravascular coagulation
    Sepsis-endotoxemia
    Preeclampsia-eclampsia
    Massive hemolysis
Association with fatty liver of pregnancy
Amniotic fluid embolism
Other causes seen in nonpregnant state
    Acute glomerulonephritis
    Subacute bacterial endocarditis
Acute postpartum renal failure

In the obstetric patient, acute renal failure appears as bilateral cortical necrosis or acute tubular necrosis. Most cases of bilateral cortical necrosis progress to chronic renal failure.[10] The condition often seems to be associated with abruptio placentae, prolonged intrauterine fetal death, and uterine hemorrhage.[6] Some authors suggest a hypercoagulable state causes this association. The extent of necrosis varies; it is most severe in the superficial cortex and frequently spares the juxtamedullary area. Extensive renovascular fibrin thrombii are seen throughout the infarcted area.[11]

Vascular hyperreactivity (with preferential cortical ischemia), glomerular changes, intraluminal obstruction, back leak of luminal contents, and abnormalities in prostaglandin metabolism have all been demonstrated in acute tubular necrosis. Which of these mechanisms is paramount in a particular type of patient is unknown. Damage is limited to the tubular cells. The extent of cell necrosis is quite variable and there may be great disparity between the severity of the lesion—frequently quite mild—and the clinical course.[12]

Most of the mortality from acute renal failure in pregnant patients is due to the severity of the underlying process rather than to the renal failure itself. Many studies have described lab tests designed to help differentiate between prerenal and parenchymal renal disease.[13] Recent research into the nature of acute renal failure has demonstrated its multifactorial nature and the possibility of lessening its severity with therapeutic maneuvers such as saline loading, mannitol, or loop diuretics. However, these laboratory models do not exactly duplicate human disease and the therapeutic interventions must be initiated within a narrow time period. Hence, we usually don't give large doses of a loop diuretic. Instead, we concentrate on the underlying disease process, using a composite of the total clinical picture.

If we believe the disease is prerenal, we try to correct the situation with appropriate fluids. Once this is done, acute renal failure should not ensue. If acute renal failure has already taken place, no known therapeutic intervention has yet been proven to reverse this process immediately. (It is also important to rule out postrenal obstruction, even though it's seen only rarely in pregnant women.)

What therapy to choose

The first and most important step in therapy is to diagnose and correct the underlying disease process. This is probably the most important factor in patient survival and it is here that the obstetrician must assume a leading role. Consider the various disease processes listed in Table 2-1 and make the appropriate diagnosis. If the patient is hypertensive, consider the diagnosis of preeclampsia. Once you have made this diagnosis, delivery is mandatory if renal function deteriorates.

If hypovolemia is present, it must be aggressively monitored and treated (Table 2-2), and the cause diagnosed and corrected. Treat serious infections with appropriate antibiotics. Usually, a broad-spectrum antibiotic should be used first, with careful adjustment of dosage if renal function is impaired. Locate and drain any abscess.

Use prothrombin time, partial thromboplastin time, platelet count, and factor VIII assay to diagnose disseminated intravascular coagulation, and correct the underlying causes. Heparin therapy is controversial; many authors prefer to concentrate entirely on the underlying cause.

If you find none of the above entities, consider the other possibilities listed in Table 2-1. If the patient is to survive, you must diagnose and control the underlying disease process.

Table 2-2. Clinical parameters for judging fluid status

Blood pressure
Pulse
Skin turgor
Mucous membrane appearance
Neck vein distention
Lung rales
Heart sounds
   Second sound in pulmonic area
   Protodiastolic gallop—S_3
Central venous pressure
   Swan-Ganz catheter if
   necessary (unusual)
Ascites
Peripheral edema
Chest x-ray for
   Heart size
   Pulmonary venous pattern
   Azygous vein dilation
   Alveolar filling pattern
   Effusions
Hematocrit changes

Adjust drug dosage and fluid administration to compensate for loss of renal function. Evaluate fluid status, electrolyte and acid-base, and the presence of uremia. The decision to dialyze usually rests on these criteria The recent trend, especially in the obstetric setting, is to dialyze early. This keeps the internal milieu as normal as possible. The clinical parameters used to determine fluid overload are listed in Table 2-2.

Electrolyte and acid-base status require careful monitoring. Be especially on guard for rapid development of hyperkalemia and acidosis, as a good deal of tissue breakdown or sequestered blood may occur as part of the underlying pathology. Although acute hyperkalemia may be treated with sodium bicarbonate, insulin and glucose, ion exchange resins, or calcium gluconate, dialysis is frequently the treatment of choice.

Once you are sure the patient requires artificial renal support, you must decide whether to choose hemo- or peritoneal dialysis. Usually, multiple factors enter into the decision (Table 2-3).

You should choose hemodialysis if the patient has had recent abdominal surgery, because peritoneal dialysis fluid tends to leak.

Table 2-3. Criteria for choosing hemo- or peritoneal dialysis

Choose hemodialysis
If the patient has had recent abdominal surgery
If the patient is obese
If there is an active pulmonary process
If the patient is massively catabolic
If access sites are not easily available
If the patient's nutritional status is poor.

Choose peritoneal dialysis
If the patient's cardiac output is inadequate
If insufficient technical support is available
If there is a bleeding diathesis
If the patient is HAA positive

Hemodialysis is also preferable for obese patients, because the peritoneal dialysis catheter may cause infection. Peritoneal dialysis is undesirable for patients with an active pulmonary process, because it tends to decrease diaphragmatic movement, and for patients who are massively catabolic, because it may not be able to keep up. Peritoneal dialysis is also indicated if blood access sites are not easily available, but not if the patient's nutritional status is poor, because of the loss of protein.

Peritoneal dialysis is a better choice if the patient's cardiac output is inadequate, since hemodialysis needs a 200 to 300 ml/minute blood flow. Because hemodialysis requires a more highly trained support group, peritoneal dialysis is indicated if technical support is inadequate. If there is a bleeding diathesis, choose peritoneal dialysis, which requires less alteration of the clotting system than hemodialysis. Finally, peritoneal dialysis is preferable if the patient is HAA positive, because there is less chance of spread to staff.

Rapidly accumulating evidence indicates that nutritional status is important not only to combat infection, repair wounds, and replace lost protein, but also to accelerate the repair process of acute tubular necrosis.[14] Early nutrition is becoming more accepted as part of the therapeutic regimen, given orally if possible, parenterally when necessary. Early dialysis, which permits control of fluids and chemistries, enables the patient to receive adequate nutrition. The patient being dialyzed has little need for the special amino acid mixes recommended by some drug manufacturers. Dialysis offers the alternative of less specific nutrition, even relatively normal meals, if the patient can manage them.

REFERENCES

1. Hayslett JP, Lynn RP: Effect of pregnancy in patients with lupus nephropathy. Kidney Int 18:207, 1980
2. Katz AI, Davison JM, Hayslett JP, et al: Pregnancy in women with kidney disease. Kidney Int 18:192, 1980
3. Singson E, Fisher K, Lindheimer MD: Acute poststreptococcal glomerulonephritis in pregnancy: Case report with an 18 year follow-up. Am J Obstet Gynecol 137:857, 1980
4. Spargo B, McCartney CP, Winemiller R: Glomerular capillary endotheliosis in toxemia of pregnancy. Arch Pathol 68:593, 1959
5. Fisher KA, Luger A, Spargo B, et al: Hypertension in pregnancy: Clinical pathological correlations and remote prognosis. Medicine. In press
6. Grunfeld J, Ganeval D, Bournerias F: Acute renal failure in pregnancy. Kidney Int 18:179, 1980
7. Robson JS, Martin AM, Ruckley VA, et al: Irreversible postpartum renal failure: A new syndrome. Q J Med 37:423, 1968
8. Schoolwerth AC, Sandler RS, Klahr S, et al: Nephrosclerosis postpartum and in women taking oral contraceptives. Arch Intern Med 136:178, 1976
9. Ferris TF: Postpartum renal insufficiency. Kidney Int 14:383, 1978
10. Kleinknecht D, Grunfeld JP, Cia-Gomez P, et al: Diagnostic procedures and long-term prognosis in bilateral renal cortical necrosis. Kidney Int 4:390, 1973
11. Spargo BH, Seymour AE, Ordonez NG: *Renal Biopsy Pathology*. New York: John Wiley & Sons, 1980, p 286
12. Lindheimer MD, Katz AI: *Kidney Function and Disease in Pregnancy*. Philadelphia: Lea & Febiger, 1977
13. Miller TR, Anderson RJ, Linas SL, et al: Urinary diagnostic indices in acute renal failure. Ann Intern Med 89:47, 1978
14. Toback FG: Amino acid enhancement of renal regeneration after acute tubular necrosis. Kidney Int 12:193, 1977

Raymond R. Schultetus, MD, PhD

Anesthetic emergencies

An expert in anesthesiology gives step-by-step directions on how to avoid serious morbidity and mortality when emergencies arise. He covers potentially fatal loss of airway control, pulmonary aspiration, toxic reactions produced by local anesthetic overdose, and paralysis due to total spinal anesthesia.

Careful adherence to good standards of practice usually results in safe anesthesia, but occasionally, in spite of reasonable precautions and good intentions, true emergencies arise. These emergencies are encountered by obstetricians as well as by anesthesiologists.

Airway control

Loss of airway control, the most acute emergency, may follow a failure to intubate the trachea after induction of general anesthesia. It also may be secondary to local anesthetic toxicity, total spinal anesthesia, or preeclampsia-eclampsia.

Assessment of the airway before surgery is the first step in preventing a potentially fatal problem.[1] Inspect the face and neck for obvious maxillofacial deformities such as a hypoplastic mandible. Palpate the neck to determine that the trachea is midline. Note jaw mobility and the size of the tongue and inspect the mouth for dentures and loose teeth. Ascertain any history of goiter, neck surgery, previous intubation, or tracheostomy. Every patient should be evaluated as though she were to be intubated.

Obesity poses special airway problems.[2] About 20% of patients near 175% of their ideal

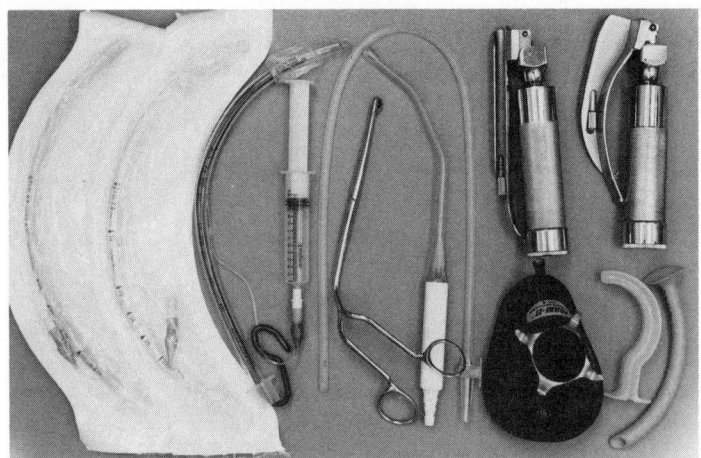

Figure 3-1. Intubation equipment includes (left to right) endotracheal tubes with stylets and syringe; Magill forceps; Yankauer suction instrument; suction catheter; laryngoscope handles with Miller (left) and MacIntosh (right) blades; and (bottom right) mask with oral and nasal airways

weight will have such problems once they are unconscious. Roughly 80% of those who exceed 300% of their ideal weight will have a tenuous airway. While the obese patient is supine and unconscious, her head and neck may become trapped in folds of adipose tissue. Pendulous breasts and chest fat may make it virtually impossible to open the mouth and insert a laryngoscope blade. The extra chest and abdominal mass compresses the thorax and increases the amount of airway pressure required to inflate the lung. For these patients and for others with tenuous airways, consider oral or nasal intubation while the patient is still awake before initiating general anesthesia.[3]

If tracheal intubation is necessary for an unconscious patient, it's mandatory to do it smoothly and rapidly. Therefore, all necessary intubation equipment should be available and ready to use (Figure 3-1). This includes:

■ Sterile cuffed endotracheal tubes with stylets. If there is time, check the cuff of the appropriate endotracheal tube (7-mm ID for most adult females) for leaks before insertion.

■ Two laryngoscope handles with blades of appropriate size (#3 MacIntosh and Miller), batteries, and bulbs. During an emergency, you will not have the time to look for spares.

■ An oxygen supply and a means for delivery such as an Ambu bag and mask, and a Yankauer suction instrument with an adequate vacuum source.

Laryngoscopy and tracheal intubation are not difficult and all physicians should be able to perform them rapidly. Although training mannequins are available, intubation skills are best developed in the operating room under the supervision of a trained laryngoscopist, using anesthetized, paralyzed patients. To facilitate laryngoscopy, place a 3- to 4-inch-thick pad under the patient's head. This thrusts the head forward into the "sniffing position," aligns the axes of the trachea, pharynx, and mouth, and makes the larynx easier to visualize. Hold the laryngoscope in the left hand and open the patient's mouth with the right (Figure 3-2, left). Insert the laryngoscope along the right side of the mouth, sweeping the tongue to the left (Figure 3-2, right). The tip of a curved blade (MacIntosh) should rest between the epiglottis and the base of the tongue. Place the tip of a straight blade (Miller) on the epiglottis, to lift it. To visualize the larynx, lift the laryngoscope at a 45° angle away from you; don't use the patient's teeth to provide leverage. Insert the endotracheal tube from the right side of the mouth—not down the center of the laryngo-

Figure 3-2. How to perform laryngoscopy and tracheal intubation. Left: Hold the laryngoscope in the left hand and open the patient's mouth with the right. Right: Insert the laryngoscope along the right side of the mouth, sweeping the tongue to the left

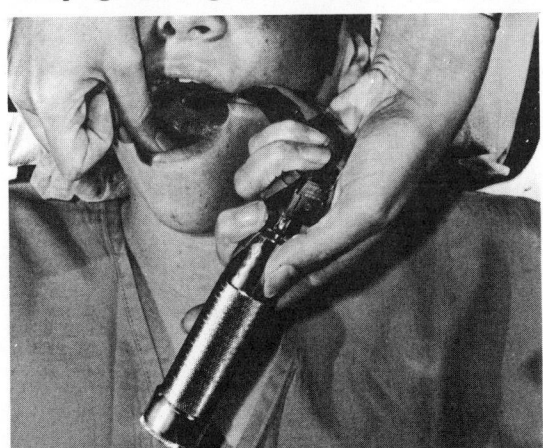
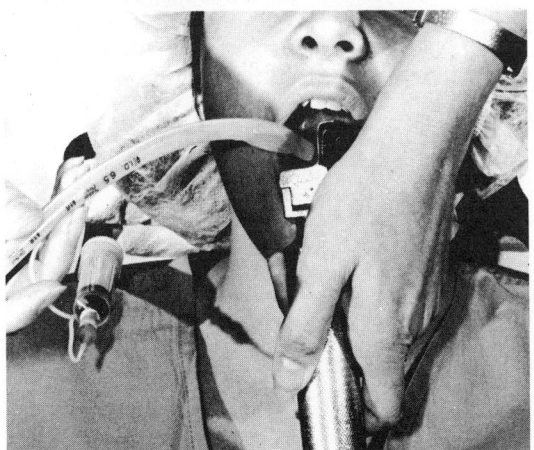

scope blade—between the vocal cords and advance it until the cuff has passed 1 to 2 cm beyond them. Inflate the cuff and auscultate the chest for bilaterally equal breath sounds.

If intubation proves impossible, use a mask to ventilate the patient. Quickly check the airway for vomitus and clear it if necessary. Apply a mask to the face with the head extended and the jaw thrust forward, and provide positive pressure ventilation (PPV) with 100% oxygen. If an unconscious patient should regurgitate during PPV, gastric contents will be forced into the trachea. However, the risk of hypoxic death outweighs the risk of pulmonary aspiration.

Because the lower esophageal sphincter has an opening pressure of approximately 18 to 20 cm H_2O, high-pressure ventilation by mask introduces air into the stomach. The resulting gastric distention further increases the likelihood of regurgitation and aspiration. Therefore, use the lowest airway pressure that will ventilate the patient adequately. Adequacy of ventilation is best judged by chest auscultation, but it can be inferred from the movement of the chest during PPV.

Application of firm posteriorly directed pressure to the cricoid cartilage by a second

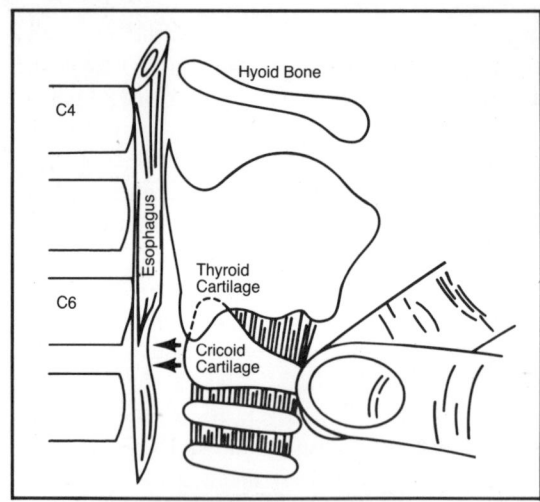

Figure 3-3. Firm, posteriorly directed pressure applied by a second person to the cricoid cartilage affords some protection from aspiration

person affords some protection from aspiration (Figure 3-3). This occludes the esophagus and prevents passive regurgitation. Because of the high pressures developed, cricoid pressure will not prevent regurgitation during active vomiting; it also could result in esophageal rupture.

If intubation cannot be accomplished and ventilation by mask is inadequate, a cricothyrotomy can sustain the patient until she can breathe or until a tracheostomy can be performed (Figure 3-4). Introduce the 12-gauge cannula into the trachea through the cricothyroid membrane and withdraw the needle. Use a 3-mm endotracheal tube adapter to connect the plastic catheter to an Ambu bag or an anesthesia machine and ventilate the patient with 100% oxygen.

Frequently, regional or local anesthesia is proposed for patients with potentially difficult airways. Remember, however, that the treatment for local anesthetic toxicity or high spinal anesthesia includes securing the airway and providing adequate ventilation, which may prove impossible. A well-planned general anesthetic with oral or nasal intubation while the patient is still awake may be a wiser choice.

Pulmonary aspiration

All unconscious patients are at risk from regurgitation and pulmonary aspiration, even those who have been fasting for 8 hours. Pregnancy imposes additional risks. Esophageal sphincter tone decreases during pregnancy—perhaps because of hormonal changes—allowing the esophageal reflux that results in the common complaint of heartburn.[4] Concurrently, intragastric pressure increases, possibly in association with increased abdominal girth.

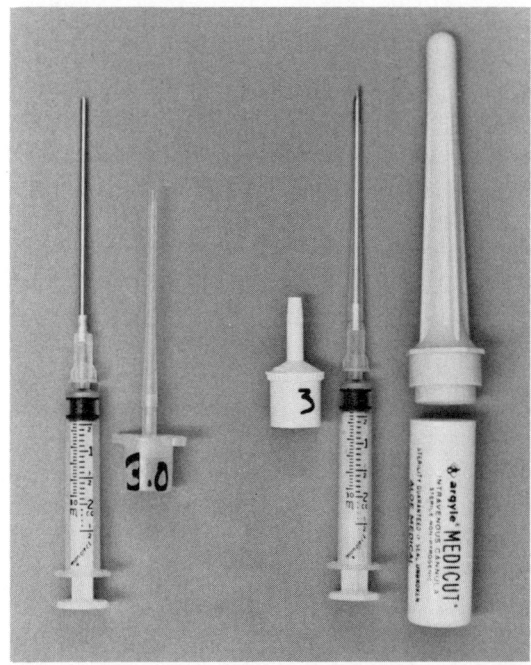

Figure 3-4. A cricothyrotomy can sustain the patient either until she can breathe or until a tracheostomy can be done. Cannula package (right) consists of needle (left), plastic catheter, and adapter

Decreased sphincter tone and increased intragastric pressure predispose the patient to regurgitation. The onset of labor increases the risk, particularly when narcotics are administered.[5] Narcotics prolong gastric emptying time and intragastric volume may quadruple as a result. When the woman in labor is obese, intragastric contents are further enlarged. As if all this weren't bad enough, patients in labor frequently have eaten and so are at extremely high risk of substantial regurgitation and severe aspiration.

To be safe, all laboring patients should be treated as though they had just eaten. To protect their lungs from reflux of gastric contents, they should never have general anesthesia without an endotracheal tube in place. If you administer inhalation or intravenous analgesia, the patient must remain alert, to protect her airway should regurgitation occur.

Acid aspiration causes chemical burns of pulmonary tissue.[6] As the aspirate pH decreases toward 1.5, the severity of the damage increases. Below pH 1.5 little additional damage is produced. Within minutes after aspiration, severe reflex bronchospasm and marked intrapulmonic shunting of blood occur. Pa_{O_2} falls to 50 to 60 torr. During the next few hours, epithelial and alveolar cells degenerate and septic necrosis begins. Hemorrhagic pulmonary edema develops and destruction of surfactant causes alveolar collapse.

The pathophysiology of the damage produced by the aspirated food depends in part upon particle size. Large particles can obstruct the large airway and cause suffocation and cardiovascular collapse. Aspiration of small particles produces hemorrhagic pneumonia, with peribronchiolar reaction centering on the particles. The pulmonary edema that results is less severe than the edema caused by acid aspiration, but hypoxemia occurs just as rapidly and may be equally profound. The aspiration of acidic food combines the effects of both types of aspiration and produces the severest lung damage.

Clinically, pulmonary aspiration of food produces tachycardia, cyanosis, dyspnea, and bronchoconstriction. Arterial oxygen tension, which falls within minutes of pulmonary aspiration, is the earliest and most reliable sign. A chest x-ray typically reveals scattered, soft, mottled, confluent densities, but these changes may lag behind clinical signs by several hours.

Because physiologic changes occur rapidly, begin therapy as soon as you suspect aspiration. Intubate the trachea to prevent further aspiration of food particles and remove any remaining material by suction. Because aspirated material rapidly disperses, prolonged or vigorous suctioning is neither useful nor recommended. Send an arterial blood sample for blood gas analysis and give supplemental oxygen.

Liquid aspirate disperses so quickly that little, if any, can be removed through the bronchoscope.[7] Do bronchoscopy only if you see large particles in the aspirate or suspect it is there. Lavage with large volumes of saline or bicarbonate is not recommended. Most studies show it produces no improvement and may actually increase the damage.[8] Solid material obstructing large airways can be removed by judicious lavage under direct vision.

Oxygen therapy and PPV improve arterial oxygenation and survival.[9] Positive end-expiratory pressure prevents airway closure and atelectasis and allows lower concentrations of inspired oxygen. The clinical course and blood gas analyses dictate what ventilatory support to use. Therapy should be directed toward keeping arterial oxygen tension above 60 torr.

Significant amounts of intravascular fluid may be lost into the lung tissue, so appropriate fluid monitoring is necessary—perhaps with a central venous or pulmonary artery catheter. Fluid therapy should be directed at maintaining normal intravascular volume and cardiac output.

There is no conclusive evidence that steroids are beneficial in aspiration therapy, although some authors continue to recommend them.[10]

Because pulmonary aspiration may introduce a wide variety of infectious organisms, prophylactic antibiotics are not indicated. Indeed, retrospective analyses of clinical courses of patients given prophylactic antibiotics showed no advantage.[11] Instead, watch for clinical signs of infection and choose antibiotics according to culture results.

Total spinal anesthesia

Injection of a large volume of local anesthetic into the subarachnoid space—which might occur with inadvertent puncture of the dura during an epidural anesthetic or cephalad migration of a smaller dose during spinal anesthesia—results in progressive and widespread neuroblockade. As anesthesia rises to the T_4

Table 3-1. Recommended maximum dosage of commonly used local anesthetic agents

Agent	Dosage limit (mg/kg)
Lidocaine (plain)	4
Lidocaine (epinephrine)	7
Bupivacaine (plain)	3
2-Chloroprocaine	10-15

Note: A 1% solution contains 10 mg/ml.

level, the intercostal muscles cease to contribute to ventilation. Although the diaphragm can maintain normal minute ventilation, the ability to cough and clear the airway is lost. A lack of sensation in the chest wall frequently gives patients a feeling that they can't breathe; however, they usually respond positively to reassurance that they are breathing adequately. As anesthesia progresses to C_4, phrenic nerves will be blocked and the diaphragm paralyzed. In addition to chest wall paralysis, total spinal anesthesia can markedly alter cardiovascular tone.

As the local anesthetic agent diffuses cephalad, it is diluted by CSF. Eventually, the local anesthetic is too diluted to penetrate large motor or sensory fibers effectively. Sympathetic fibers, arising from preganglionic cells located in spinal cord segments T_1 through L_4, are smaller and may still be affected. This results in a sympathetic blockade usually at least two segments higher than the sensory. Thus, spinal anesthesia to a sensory level of T_4 could occur concurrently with a sympathetic blockade to T_1. Since the sympathetic nervous system maintains vascular tone, a total sympathetic blockade allows venous pooling of blood.

Sympathetic cardiac accelerator fibers, which maintain heart rate, are found at spinal cord levels T_1 through T_4. High spinal anesthesia blocks these fibers and produces bradycardia. The marked decrease in cardiac output caused by reduced venous return and heart rate produces severe hypotension, which can result in medullary ischemia and respiratory arrest.

Total spinal anesthesia requires adequate ventilation with oxygen and cardiovascular support. Usually, the patient needs to be intubated to ensure adequate ventilation and to secure the airway against aspiration. Circulatory support involves displacing the uterus to the left to relieve aortocaval compression, raising the legs to improve venous return, and administering fluid therapy and drugs to restore peripheral vascular tone. Ephedrine is best as the first-line vasopressor. It produces both vasoconstriction and cardiac stimulation and restores cardiac output and blood pressure without decreasing uterine blood flow. Use normal saline, Ringer's lactate, or albumin to expand intravascular volume. Because several liters of fluid may be required, don't give fluids containing dextrose for resuscitation. The infusion of even very small amounts of dextrose can produce neonatal hypoglycemia.[12]

The incidence of total spinal anesthesia is low (less than 0.1%), yet it remains a serious potential complication of epidural, spinal, and caudal anesthesia.[13]

Toxic reactions to local anesthetics

Allergic reactions to local anesthetics are rare; toxic reactions to a high plasma concentration of local anesthetic occur more frequently. The incidence of seizures induced by anesthetics during epidural blockade is estimated at 0.2%.[14] High blood concentrations result from intravascular injection, rapid uptake from highly vascular tissues, or, simply, too high a dosage. Early signs of toxicity include nervousness, dizziness, tinnitus, and tremors. The patient may be confused and have blurred vision and nystagmus. As drug levels increase, tonic-clonic seizures occur. Drug-induced CNS depression may closely follow an initial period of excitation. At high blood levels, you may see respiratory arrest and cardiovascular depression with hypotension, bradycardia, and cardiac arrest. Some early signs of toxicity (nervousness, tremor, and headache) may be difficult to distinguish from the effects of epinephrine, often used in conjunction with local anesthetic agents.

Seizures induced by local anesthetics are generally of short duration (usually less than 1 minute), because of the rapidity with which these drugs are redistributed. To treat, maintain the airway and give oxygen. In animal studies, this therapy alone markedly reduces the morbidity and mortality from such seizures.[15] Cardiovascular depression requires treatment with fluids and vasopressors. The use of benzodiazepines (2.5 to 5 mg, IV) and short-acting barbiturates (50 to 100 mg, IV) to terminate seizure activity is controversial because such drugs may depress the cardiovascular system further and delay return to consciousness. Terminating a seizure with these agents, however, may permit effective ventilation, restoring cardiovascular stability and improving cerebral oxygenation. Giving the muscle relaxant succinylcholine (20 to 40 mg, IV) to produce paralysis allows ventilation during a seizure. Succinylcholine does not depress the myocardium or alter consciousness, nor does it block cortical seizures. However, muscle relaxants should never be used unless adequate ventilation can be assured after paralysis has been induced.

Preventing toxicity is preferable to treating it. Inject local anesthetic agents slowly and check frequently for blood, to avoid intravascular injection. Follow dosage limits (see Table 3-1). The limits refer to the maximum for a single injection. With repeated injections, the maximum is lower, because of the long half-life of most local anesthetics and the resultant cumulative effect. Additional dosage corrections are required to allow for a patient's physical condition and any special problems, such as renal or hepatic disease, that alter metabolism and excretion. Finally, local anesthesia should never be used unless resuscitation equipment is available.

To avoid serious morbidity and mortality, you must respond quickly and appropriately to all the emergencies cited. This chapter is not meant to be an exhaustive treatise on therapy. It is designed to alert readers to potentially serious complications and stimulate them to practice old skills and learn new ones.

REFERENCES

1. Ament R: A systematic approach to the difficult intubation. Anesthesiol Rev 5(7):12, 1978
2. Lee JJ, Larson RH, Buckley JJ, et al: Airway maintenance in the morbidly obese. Anesthesiol Rev 7(1):33, 1980
3. Donlon JV Jr: Anesthetic management of patients with compromised airways. Anesthesiol Rev 7(2):22, 1980
4. Brock-Utne JG, Dow TBG, Dimopoulos GE, et al: Gastric and lower oesophageal sphincter (LOS) pressures in early pregnancy. Br J Anaesth 53:381, 1981
5. Roberts RB, Shirley MA: Reducing the risk of acid aspiration during cesarean section. Anesth Analg 53(6):859, 1974
6. Wynne JW, Modell JH: Respiratory aspiration of stomach contents. Ann Intern Med 87:466, 1977
7. Hamelberg W, Bosomworth PP: Aspiration pneumonitis: Experimental studies and clinical observations. Anesth Analg 43:669, 1964
8. Taylor G, Pryse-Davies J: Evaluation of endotracheal steroid therapy in acid pulmonary aspiration syndrome (Mendelson's syndrome). Anesthesiology 29:17, 1968
9. Cameron JL, Sebor J, Anderson RP, et al: Aspiration pneumonia. Results of treatment by positive-pressure ventilation in dogs. J Surg Res 8:447, 1968
10. Chapman RL Jr, Downs JB, Modell JH, et al: The ineffectiveness of steroid therapy in treating aspiration of hydrochloric acid. Arch Surg 108:858, 1974
11. Cameron JL, Mitchell WH, Zuidema GD: Aspiration pneumonia. Clinical outcome following documented aspiration. Arch Surg 106:49, 1973
12. Knepp NB, Shelley WC, Kumer S, et al: Effects on newborn of hydration with glucose in patients undergoing cesarean section with regional anesthesia. Lancet 1:645, 1980
13. Dawkins CJM: An analysis of the complications of epidural and caudal block. Anaesthesia 24:554, 1969
14. Kandel PF, Spoerel WE, Kinch RAH: Continuous epidural analgesia for labour and delivery. Review of 1000 cases. Can Med Assoc J 95:947, 1966
15. Feinstein MB, Lenard W, Mathios J: The antagonism of local anesthetic induced convulsions by the benzodiazepine derivative diazepam. Arch Int Pharmacodyn Ther 187:144, 1970

Robert H. Hayashi, MD

Responding to cardiorespiratory complications

The author describes heart and lung alterations during pregnancy and specific gynecologic procedures. Then he tells how to deal with acute pulmonary edema, reversal of intracardiac shunt, acute myocardial infarction, arrhythmia, adult respiratory distress syndrome, and the syndrome that follows evacuation of molar pregnancy.

Cardiorespiratory complications are rare in ob/gyn patients. All the more reason to stress the signs and symptoms, so the clinician can be ready to treat the occasional emergency. I'll begin by reviewing how pregnancy and various gynecologic situations alter the cardiorespiratory system. Then I will move on to management of several common clinical entities (Table 4-1).

Cardiorespiratory changes

Normal pregnant women often complain of excessive fatigue, shortness of breath, and peripheral edema. These complaints should not be ignored, because they are also those of patients in early congestive heart failure. The placenta provides a large arteriovenous shunt that results in a hyperdynamic cardiovascular state. Total peripheral vascular resistance decreases and midtrimester blood pressures often go below prepregnancy levels. Blood volume (proportionately more plasma volume than RBC volume) increases by 20% to 100% in midtrimester. Cardiac output increases by 30% to 50%, mainly as a result of increased stroke volume (20% to 40%); heart rate increases only 10% to 15%. Early postpartum, extravascular fluid volume rapidly shifts into the vascular compartment, requiring cardiac output 60% above prepregnancy levels.

Decreased muscular tone of the chest wall during pregnancy increases the anterior-posterior and lateral diameters of the chest, with elevation and flattening of the diaphragm. The pregnant woman's heart rotates laterally, so that the point of maximal impulse shifts to the left and the electrical axis of the ECG also shifts to the left by about 15°. The ECG can also show T-wave inversion and a Q wave in lead III. The changes in the chest cavity contribute decreased functional residual capacity and increased tidal volume. Only the vital capacity is unchanged. The respiratory system is not particularly stressed in pregnancy. In fact, it becomes superefficient.

In gynecologic patients, acute cardiorespiratory complications are likely to occur during the intra- and postoperative periods. For example, older patients may have acute myocardial ischemia or heart damage. Hemorrhagic shock resulting in adult respiratory distress syndrome, aspiration pneumonitis, and pulmonary emboli are potential complications of gynecologic surgery.

Heart problems

Acute pulmonary edema. Obstetric patients develop pulmonary edema in several ways. The cardiac patient with rheumatic mitral valve disease may have acute left ventricular failure. Patients are likely to go into heart failure when the changes of pregnancy demand increased cardiac output, that is, in midpregnancy, late in the second stage of labor, and immediately postpartum. As left atrial pressure increases, myocardial failure raises pulmonary venous and capillary pressures. When pulmonary intravascular pressure rises above colloid osmotic pressure (COP), free fluid leaves the vascular tree and enters the alveoli and terminal bronchioles—producing pulmonary edema.[1]

Patients with severe preeclampsia or eclampsia may develop pulmonary edema. Their total peripheral vascular resistance may rise and increase cardiac workload; their COP may fall because of hypoalbuminemia; and those with decreased intravascular volume may be easily overloaded when IV fluids are administered. Those being treated for premature labor with sympathomimetic agents, with and without corticosteroids, are also at risk for pulmonary edema.[2,3] The cause in this case is unclear, but the edema usually follows prolonged therapy and substantial volumes of IV fluids. Pulmonary edema has been reported when large volumes of fluid are infused, when there is no heart failure.[4]

Patients with acute pulmonary edema may have suffocating dyspnea, tachypnea, anxiety, and labored breathing. Physical examination shows diffuse rales and frothy, possibly blood-tinged, sputum. Chest x-rays usually show diffuse or perihilar infiltrates in both lung fields.

Treat acute pulmonary edema by having the patient sit up, give 5 to 15 mg IM morphine to relieve anxiety, and administer oxygen by mask. Oxygen by positive pressure raises intrapulmonary pressure and decreases pulmonary venous return to the heart—this could be an added benefit. Give 40 mg furosemide (Lasix) as a slow IV injection, and repeat in 15 to 20 minutes, if necessary. This rapidly acting diuretic has the additional benefit of decreasing venomotor tone to promote peripheral venous pooling.[5]

Consider rapid digitalizing of the cardiac patient to enhance myocardial function. But use digitalis with caution, if at all, for patients who have recently been given sympathomimetic drugs for premature labor. Such patients tend to be hypokalemic. Digoxin at 0.5 mg IV will produce rapid results. Give six additional doses of digoxin, 0.125 mg IV, at 2-hour intervals for full digitalization. If left heart failure is associated with acute hypertension, lower the blood pressure to lessen the cardiac afterload work. You can inject hydralazine (Apresoline hydrochloride) intermittently, 5 to 10 mg IV, or in a constant infusion (50 mg in 500 ml D_5W), to lower the diastolic pressure to 90 to 110 mm Hg. Obtain hourly readings of urine output, frequent serum electrolyte levels, and periodic arterial blood gases and ECGs. Correct any hypokalemia, particularly in patients treated for premature labor.

If flow-directed catheters (Swan-Ganz) are available for monitoring pulmonary capillary wedge pressure (PCWP), use them. This type of monitoring can provide a clue to the patho-

Table 4-1. Management of ob/gyn cardiorespiratory complications

Pulmonary edema
- Have patient sitting.
- Administer morphine, 5 to 15 mg IM.
- Give IPPB with O_2.
- Infuse furosemide, 40 mg IV, slowly (may repeat in 15 to 20 minutes).
- Prescribe digoxin, 0.5 mg IV, then 0.125 mg IV q 2 h for total of six doses, but not if patient is hypokalemic.
- Treat underlying conditions.

Reversal of intracardiac shunt
- Identify patient at risk.
- Have IVs in both arms and blood ready at delivery.
- Replace any blood or volume loss quickly.
- Infuse dopamine, 10 µg/kg/minute; increase by 1 to 4 µg/kg/minute q 15 m.

Ventricular ectopic beats
- Give lidocaine IV bolus of 50-100 mg, approximately 1 mg/kg (may repeat).
- Follow with continuous infusion, 4 mg/minute, and taper over 24 hours.
- *Or* give procainamide, 0.2-1.0 gm IV, very slowly.
- Treat ventricular fibrillation by dc defibrillator (300-400 W/second).

Adult respiratory distress syndrome
- Give PEEP ventilation.
- Maintain strict intake-output fluid balance.
- Use diuretics cautiously.
- Treat underlying conditions aggressively.

physiology of the edema. COP measurements may indicate whether an albumin infusion along with furosemide might be beneficial.

Once the edema subsides, the specific obstetric and medical problems will dictate care. Serial measurements of total pulmonary vital capacity are useful for following patients who risk congestive heart failure.[6]

Reversal of intracardiac shunt. Certain congenital heart defects are associated with intracardiac left-to-right shunts: atrial and ventricular septal defects, Eisenmenger syndrome, and tetralogy of Fallot. About two-thirds of maternal deaths associated with these conditions occur around delivery.[7] Excessive blood loss or decreased peripheral vascular resistance may reverse the left-to-right shunt, causing a bypass of the lungs. Hypoxemia will quickly ensue. The best management of these patients is preventive. Have large-bore IV catheters in both arms, and blood in the delivery suite, to correct excessive blood loss quickly. Avoid conduction anesthesia and the supine hypotension syndrome.

If a shunt reversal occurs, expand the circulating volume as quickly as possible and consider using a peripheral vasoconstrictor to increase left heart afterload pressure. If you try a dopamine infusion (800 µg/ml concentration), begin at 10 µg/kg/minute and increase by 1 to 4 µg/kg/minute every 15 minutes until the patient is normotensive. At this dosage, the drug will increase cardiac output and peripheral resistance. Once the shunt reversal has occurred, survival is low.

Acute myocardial infarction. One in 10,000 deliveries is complicated by acute myocardial infarction. The disorder is more frequent when older women have gynecologic procedures. Anterior chest pain and ECG changes will clinch the diagnosis. Because myocardial ischemia is manifested by exaggerated inverted T waves, the ECG changes may include some of the following (Figure 4-1): tall T waves that indicate subendocardial ischemia (A); inverted T waves that indicate epicardial ischemia (B); RST-segment depression that indicates subendocardial injury (C); and RST-segment elevation that indicates epicardial injury (D). ECG death is usually the equivalent of biologic death and results in QS waves in the lead facing the area of transmural infarction (E).[8]

Management of pregnant patients with an infarction would include oxygen, analgesics, intensive care, monitoring for arrhythmias, but no anticoagulants. The gynecologic patient might be given anticoagulants, depending on whether or not she is postoperative. These decisions should be made with the attending cardiologist.

Cardiac arrhythmia. Pregnant patients are more prone than nonpregnant women to episodes of paroxysmal tachycardia. A healthy woman can tolerate these episodes, but carotid sinus stimulation, Valsalva maneuver, or

Figure 4-1. Characteristic ECG forms of ischemic events*

A — Subendocardial ischemia
B — Epicardial ischemia
C — Subendocardial injury
D — Epicardial injury
E — Electrical death

A—Tall T waves.
B—Inverted coved T waves.
C—RST-segment depression.
D—RST-segment elevation.
E—QS wave.

*Adapted from Santinga JT.[8]

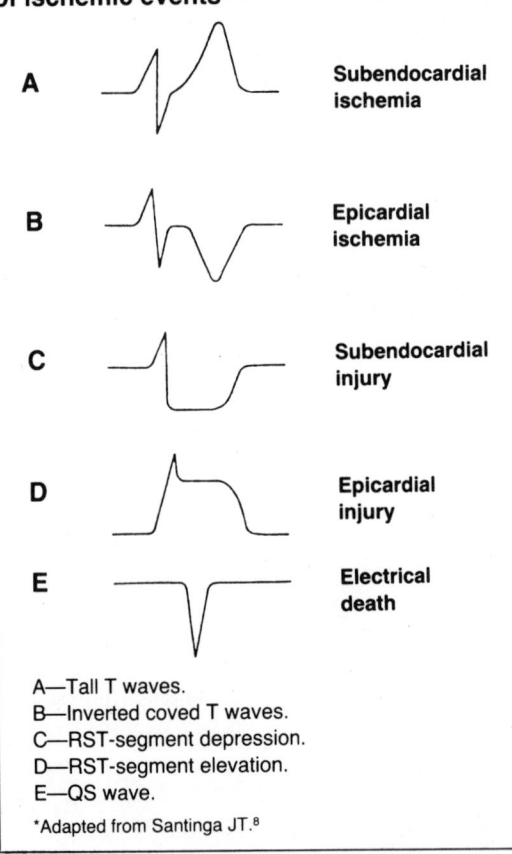

digitalis or quinidine may help. If the patient has any hemodynamic embarrassment from the supraventricular tachycardia, and the vagal stimulation maneuvers fail, use direct current (dc) cardioversion. This is effective and safe during pregnancy.[9] Use the synchronizer circuit on the dc defibrillator at the low-energy level (20 W/second).

During early labor, consider using antiarrhythmia agents if warning arrhythmias appear on the ECG (frequent premature ventricular contractions, R-on-T phenomenon, multifocality, bigeminy, or short bursts of ventricular tachycardia).[10] Risk of hypoxemia or hypotension is substantial in peripartum.

Lidocaine effectively controls ventricular ectopic activity if prompt treatment is necessary.[11] Give an IV bolus of lidocaine, 10 to 100 mg (approximately 1 mg/kg), rapidly. This dose may be repeated every 3 to 5 minutes until the dysrhythmia is suppressed (doses in excess of 300 mg approach toxic levels). Follow bolus doses of lidocaine immediately with continuous infusion of 20 to 50 µg/kg/minute (or 1 to 4 mg/minute in the 70-kg patient). For example, begin a 4 mg/minute infusion immediately (1 gm lidocaine in 500 ml D_5W) after the bolus, and gradually taper during the next 24 hours.[12] Some patients will respond to depressants such as procainamide (Pronestyl), quinidine, or disopyramide (Norpace) when lidocaine has failed.[10] The usual IV dose of procainamide hydrochloride is 0.2 to 1.0 gm and should be given very slowly at a rate not in excess of 25 to 50 mg/minute. For ventricular fibrillation, use the dc defibrillator at 300 to 400 W/second.

Atrial fibrillation in a pregnant woman with rheumatic heart disease places her at risk for pulmonary embolus (23%) and heart failure.[13] Try to restore normal sinus rhythm, administer digitalis to slow the ventricular response, and then give a maintenance dose of quinidine (0.2 to 0.3 gm orally every 6 to 8 hours). If atrial fibrillation persists, use dc cardioversion. If atrial fibrillation persists or recurs, seriously consider long-term anticoagulation.

When the lung is involved

Adult respiratory distress syndrome (ARDS). This serious and potentially fatal pulmonary disease may complicate a variety of obstetric and gynecologic conditions: amniotic fluid embolism, aspiration, severe preeclampsia, eclampsia, massive fluid infusions, sepsis, and intra-abdominal or pelvic abscesses.[14] ARDS has been well recognized in association with massive trauma and shock.

Progressive respiratory distress and severe hypoxemia, relatively refractory to high inspired oxygen tension, characterize the syndrome. Chest x-rays show diffuse infiltrates.

The picture is similar to that of pulmonary edema, except that the patchy or fluffy infiltrates involve the entire lung field. The alveolar-capillary membrane becomes increasingly permeable, and progressive interstitial and alveolar edema results. You can differentiate cardiac from noncardiac pulmonary edema by

Table 4-2. Aspiration pneumonitis

- Perform endotracheal suction if aspiration is noted.
- Infuse with hydrocortisone, 1 gm IV, at once and q 4 h.
- Give IPPB with O_2.
- Monitor arterial blood gases (patient may need intubation or tracheostomy).
- Administer aminophylline, 250 to 500 mg in 50 ml of D_5W, over 20 minutes to counteract bronchospasm.
- Consider antibiotics to prevent secondary infections.

determining the PCWP with a flow-directed catheter. In ARDS, the pulmonary artery pressures and pulmonary vascular resistance may be elevated, but the PCWP remains low or normal; in cardiogenic pulmonary edema, the PCWP is elevated.[15]

To manage ARDS, support cardiovascular and respiratory functions and treat underlying or associated conditions. Positive end-expiratory pressure (PEEP) ventilation has become the key in the therapy. PEEP increases arterial oxygenation by increasing lung volumes and decreasing intrapulmonary shunting. The goal is to maintain arterial oxygenation of at least 60 torr. This generally requires a tidal volume of 10 to 20 cc/kg and a PEEP level of 5 to 35 cm H_2O.[15] Balance the intake and output of fluids. Use diuretics with caution, and give antibiotics and packed red blood cell transfusions as needed. The use of steroids has been controversial. Again, aggressive management of the underlying condition is critical to recovery.

Postevacuation of molar pregnancy syndrome. Acute respiratory insufficiency in the early postevacuation period among patients with a uterus of 16 weeks or greater has a reported incidence of 27%.[16] The syndrome is characterized by tachycardia, tachypnea, and hypoxemia.[17] Chest x-rays demonstrate patchy or fluffy, bilateral, pulmonary infiltrates and, sometimes, a concomitant pleural effusion. Contributing factors include deportation of trophoblastic tissue, hyperthyroidism, fluid overload, dilutional anemia, preeclampsia, and general anesthesia.[16,17] Before evacuating a mole, document blood gases for baseline study. Watch fluids in the pre-, intra-, and postoperative periods and carefully moni-

Table 4-3. Pulmonary embolus

- Give 5,000 to 10,000 units of heparin IV initially and then repeat every 4 to 6 hours. Maintain whole blood clotting time at two to three times normal or the activated PTT at one and a half to two times normal.
- Prescribe constant infusion of approximately 1,000 units of heparin per hour as acceptable alternative. Monitor the same way.
- Watch for hemorrhagic complications.
- Order O_2 and mild sedation.
- If repeated embolization occurs while patient is on anticoagulant therapy, surgically interrupt inferior vena cava and possibly left ovarian vein.

tor CVP. Treat aggressively any underlying condition such as hyperthyroidism, preeclampsia, or anemia. Use oxygen, sedation, and diuretics as needed. The syndrome is uniformly transient, with good outcome, but patients have been reported at risk of later having invasive mole or choriocarcinoma.[7]

Tables 4-2 to 4-4 give management protocols for treating aspiration pneumonitis, pulmonary embolus, and amniotic fluid embolus. These entities have been discussed in detail in an earlier chapter.[18]

Table 4-4. Amniotic fluid embolus

- Have patient sitting.
- Inject morphine, 5 to 15 mg IM.
- Give IPPB with O_2.
- Give aminophylline, 250 to 500 mg in 50 ml D_5W, over 20 minutes.
- Prescribe digoxin, 0.5 mg IV, then 0.125 mg IV q 2 h for six doses.
- Order hydrocortisone, 1 gm IV; follow with 250 mg q 4 h.
- Compress uterus to control atony.
- Make judicious use of blood transfusion therapy.
- Combat coagulopathy with fresh frozen plasma or cryoprecipitate.

REFERENCES

1. Rackow EC, Fein IA, Leppo A: Colloid osmotic pressure as a prognostic indicator of pulmonary edema and mortality in the critically ill. Chest 72:709, 1979
2. Jacobs MM, Knight AB, Arias F: Maternal pulmonary edema resulting from betamimetic and glucocorticoid therapy. Obstet Gynecol 56:56, 1980
3. Katz M, Robertson PA, Creasy RK: Cardiovascular complications associated with terbutaline treatment for preterm labor. Am J Obstet Gynecol 139:605, 1981
4. Stein L, Beraud J, Cavanilles J, et al: Pulmonary edema during fluid infusion in the absence of heart failure. JAMA 229:65, 1974
5. Dikshit K, Vyden JK, Forrester JS, et al: Renal and extrarenal hemodynamic effects of furosemide in congestive heart failure after acute myocardial infarction. N Engl J Med 288:1087, 1973
6. Kannel WB, Seidman JM, Fercho W, et al: Vital capacity and congestive heart failure: The Framingham study. Circulation 49:1160, 1974
7. Conradsson TB, Werko L: Management of heart disease in pregnancy. Prog Cardiovasc Dis 16:407, 1974
8. Santinga JT: Electrocardiographic diagnosis of anterior myocardial infarction. Univ Mich Med Ctr J 40:20, 1974
9. Schroeder JS, Harrison DC: Repeated cardioversion during pregnancy. Am J Cardiol 27:445, 1971
10. Myerburg RJ, Besozzi MC: Decisions in the treatment of ventricular ectopic activity. JAMA 240:476, 1978
11. Lie KI, Wellens JH, van Capelle FJ, et al: Lidocaine in the prevention of primary ventricular fibrillation: A double blind, randomized study of 212 consecutive patients. N Engl J Med 291:1324, 1974
12. Collinsworth KA, Kalman SM, Harrison DC: The clinical pharmacology of lidocaine as an antiarrhythmic drug. Circulation 50:1217, 1974
13. Mendelson CL: Disorders of the heart during pregnancy. Am J Obstet Gynecol 72:1268, 1956
14. Andersen HF, Lynch JP, Johnson TRB Jr: Adult respiratory distress syndrome in obstetrics and gynecology. Obstet Gynecol 55:291, 1980
15. Zapol WM, Snider MT: Pulmonary hypertension in severe acute respiratory failure. N Engl J Med 296:476, 1977
16. Cotton DB, Bernstein SG, Read JA, et al: Hemodynamic observations in evacuation of molar pregnancy. Am J Obstet Gynecol 138:6, 1980
17. Twiggs LB, Morrow CP, Schlaerth JB: Acute pulmonary complications of molar pregnancy. Am J Obstet Gynecol 135:189, 1979
18. Huff RW, Hayashi RH: Emergencies in obstetric patients: Difficulties in breathing. Contemp Ob/Gyn 11:54, Jan 1978

Gail V. Anderson, MD
Alan Ball, PA-C

Managing acute abdominal problems in pregnancy

This chapter describes the symptoms of the most common acute conditions and tells how best to manage them, particularly during pregnancy and in the period following delivery.

Assuming that a patient's abdominal symptoms are a result of pregnancy may delay diagnosis and treatment of an acute abdominal crisis, with catastrophic consequences.

The approach to any surgical problem of a pregnant or puerperal patient should be the same as for a nonpregnant patient, with prompt surgical intervention when indicated. The risk of precipitating labor with diagnostic laparotomy is negligible, provided unnecessary surgical maneuvers are avoided.[1] Spontaneous abortion is most likely to occur if surgery is performed before 16 weeks' gestation or when there is peritonitis and fluid in the peritoneal cavity.

Diagnosing appendicitis

Appendicitis is the most common acute abdominal problem during pregnancy. It occurs slightly more often in the second trimester than in the first and third. Signs during pregnancy are fewer and more limited.

The acute focal stage begins with an obstructive insult of the appendiceal lumen that is traceable to hypertrophied submucosal follicles following a viral infection (60%), fecalith (35%), foreign body (4%), or stricture (0.5%). The patient feels visceral pain in the periumbilical or epigastric areas.[2] As mucus accumulates and is turned to pus by bacterial and leukocytic action, distention, edema, and ulceration proceed to acute suppurative appendicitis. Pain is confined to the right lower quadrant in nonpregnant patients and those in early pregnancy. Venous distention and obstruction, ischemia, and bacterial invasion of the wall of the appendix cause irritation of the overlying parietal peritoneum and produce point tenderness.

Whether the pain is in the right iliac fossa depends on gestation. The enlarging uterus displaces the cecum and appendix upward, laterally, and often posteriorly. At term, the appendix is well above the iliac crest. The long axis changes counterclockwise from a downward to an upward direction.[3]

Once peritonitis sets in, in the wake of perforation, the pregnant patient may be moribund within 24 hours. During late second and third trimesters, the bulk of the uterus displaces the omentum upward, preventing "walling off" of the infection and allowing it to disseminate faster. The presence of pus after perforation causes irritability in the uterus, which forms the medial border of any appendiceal abscess or local peritonitis. This process induces preterm labor. With infarction, gangrene, or peritonitis, fetal mortality increases markedly.

You can elicit Alder's sign (fixed tenderness) by finding the point of maximal tenderness on the abdominal wall and turning the patient onto her left side without changing the position or pressure of the examining fingers. The pain produced by the pressure will be reduced if the lesion is intrauterine and has fallen away from the examining fingers. If the pain is unaltered, the lesion is extrauterine. A few patients will not perceive the pain if the appendix is not in contact with the parietal peritoneum.

Leukocytosis is not helpful. During pregnancy, there is a physiologic increase in white blood cells to 11,000 to 16,000 per ml. On x-ray, the most frequent sign is air-fluid levels or gaseous distention of the cecum or the adjacent small bowel, interpreted as a local adynamic ileus. (While x-rays of pregnant patients should be avoided, particularly during the first trimester, they sometimes must be done to establish the diagnosis.) Convex lumbar scoliosis, psoas obliteration, and appendicolith are also seen.[4] None of these is pathognomonic for appendicitis.

It is helpful to differentiate acute appendicitis from acute salpingitis (rare in pregnancy). Nausea and vomiting accompany both but are more frequent in appendicitis. The tenderness in salpingitis is usually bilateral and is accompanied by a higher temperature elevation (103°F) than is acute unruptured appendicitis. (100°F). Guarding or rebound tenderness is less likely in salpingitis and bowel sounds are usually normal.

Acute pyelonephritis, the most serious medical complication of pregnancy, is frequently confused with appendicitis when it involves the right side. Chills and fever (103° to 104°F) accompanied by costovertebral angle pain are the most common initial symptoms. Chills seldom herald the onset of appendicitis and the temperature is rarely as high as 103°F. Frequency, dysuria, nausea, and vomiting are common in pyelonephritis. As a rule, there is no abdominal muscle rigidity, while in acute appendicitis, local rigidity is often present. An uncentrifuged urine sample that shows pyuria and bacteriuria is usually sufficient to incriminate the urinary tract as the source of the problem.[5,6]

Significant transient reversible renal dysfunction, possibly caused by endotoxemia, has been reported in a fifth of pyelonephritis cases. Exercise care when using nephrotoxic drugs and any drug excreted by the kidneys, if transient dysfunction becomes evident.

Urolithiasis is less common than pyelonephritis as a cause of abdominal pain in pregnancy. Pain is usually on the right side. Urolithiasis is differentiated from pyelonephritis by urinary findings. Pain associated with renal stones radiates to the groin or genitalia. However, if symptoms of pain referable to the kidney persist (especially on the left side), renal stones should be considered.

Ovarian cysts

Complications of ovarian cysts during pregnancy and the puerperium are second to appendicitis in frequency. Torsion occurs in one pregnancy in a thousand and spontaneous rupture in approximately 2% of all ovarian cysts.[7,8]

Ovarian cysts—and sometimes normal ovaries and tubes—may become ischemic because of torsion resulting from pressure and displacement during pregnancy and labor. Typically, there is acute lower abdominal pain on the affected side. Crampy, intermittent discomfort may occur initially if torsion is partial or self-limited, and patients may have recurrent episodes. The pain may radiate to the flank or thigh. Vomiting is frequently an early manifestation of torsion; in appendicitis it occurs later. A tender mass may be palpable in the left or right lower quadrant, adjacent to the uterus.

Acute rupture of an ovarian cyst is more common in the pregnant than the nonpregnant woman. The initial symptom is usually acute severe pain; there may be some evidence of peritonitis. Acute peritonitis results from rupture of a dermoid cyst, and subacute granulomatous peritonitis and dense adhesions result from continued leakage.

Elective operations on the ovary should be deferred until the 16th week or after, because of the increased incidence of spontaneous abortion before that time. However, ovarian cysts large enough to be discovered during pregnancy should be removed soon after discovery because the risk of complications outweighs the risk of laparotomy.[9]

Tubo-ovarian abscess and salpingitis

Pregnancy and salpingitis or tubo-ovarian abscess rarely coexist. It is generally safer to seek another diagnosis.

Distinguishing between salpingitis and tubo-ovarian abscess with impending rupture is the principal problem in managing pelvic inflammatory disease. Salpingitis usually is accompanied by a vaginal discharge. There may be a history of infection by intercourse; a recent gynecologic or contraceptive procedure; a latent focal flare-up or nearby focus (such as appendicitis); or spread of bacteria from another focus of infection via the blood or lymphatic system.

The gonococcus is the usual cause of acute salpingitis; staphylococcal, streptococcal, or *Escherichia coli* infections occur less often. Patients with acute salpingitis usually consult a physician later than those with acute appendicitis. Symptom onset is closely related to the menstrual cycle.

The initial complaint is usually pelvic pain, often progressing from chronic to severe. In most instances, unruptured abscesses "point" to the pelvis and are managed quite successfully by colpotomy or proctotomy and insertion of a larger "dog-ear" drain into the abscess cavity. However, an unruptured abscess, felt as a unilateral or bilateral tender pelvic mass, not responding to conservative management, may rupture into the peritoneal cavity. Rupture is heralded by a sudden increase in pain, rapidly followed by generalized peritonitis, manifested by spiking temperature, tachycardia, and marked abdominal tenderness with muscle spasm. Shock will follow if ileus treatment is not instituted promptly. Culdocentesis frequently yields purulent material. *E. coli* is recovered most frequently and may be associated with β-hemolytic streptococci, *Staphylococcus aureus*, *Klebsiella*, *Proteus*, or *Bacteroides fragilis*. There is no place for "conservative" (nonsurgical) management of a ruptured tubo-ovarian abscess.[10]

Major complications stem directly from a delay in treatment and incomplete operation.[11] Patients with tubo-ovarian abscess seldom become pregnant and the abscess continues to be a source of ill health. Therefore, complete removal of uterus, tubes, and ovaries is advisable.[12] Insertion of rubber drains through an open vaginal cuff to allow thorough drainage of the operative site further decreases the chance of complications.

Before and during surgery, give colloids and crystalloids IV, along with blood and plasma, to maintain adequate volume, as indicated by estimated blood loss, hematocrit, urine output, urine specific gravity, clinical state of hydration, and central venous pressure (CVP). Monitoring the CVP is the best way to maintain hydration and oxygen-carrying capabilities and prevent fluid overload.

Give large doses of hydrocortisone preoperatively and 24 hours postoperatively to severely ill patients or those debilitated by prolonged illness or who have vascular collapse secondary to sepsis. It is not necessary to taper the dose of hydrocortisone or to give ACTH when steroids are administered for such a short period.

Acute intestinal obstruction

Adhesions are the most common cause of intestinal obstruction in both the general and pregnant populations. Incarcerated hernias and bowel neoplasms are the next most common causes in the general population, and volvulus and intussusception in pregnancy. Because the most frequent causes of adhesions are appendectomies and gynecologic procedures, consider obstruction in symptomatic patients who have had abdominal surgery.[13] Bowel obstruction is an unusual complication during pregnancy, but delay in diagnosis can lead to episodes of maternal hypoxia and hypotension that can be fatal for the fetus.

Adhesions are most likely to precipitate obstruction during three time periods: in the fourth to fifth month, when the uterus changes from a pelvic to an abdominal position, causing traction on previous adhesions; in the eighth to ninth month, when the fetal head descends into the pelvis; and in the period immediately after delivery, when a sudden change in uterine size drastically alters the relation of adhesions to the surrounding bowel. According to Goldthrop, most cases of intestinal obstruction secondary to adhesions occur during the first pregnancy after an operation.[13] The average time between symptoms and hospital admission is 3.5 days and between admission and operation is 2.8 days.[14]

Diagnosis is based on a classic triad of colicky abdominal pain, vomiting increasing in frequency and amount, and absolute constipation. Remember, constipation is common in pregnancy—obstipation is not.[15]

The degree and suddenness of obstruction govern onset and severity of symptoms. An obstruction high up in the small bowel will produce early symptoms of frequent, violent vomiting associated with pain and shock. Distention is not an early feature and the vomitus will be green and bilious unless obstruction is proximal to the ampulla of Vater. Symptoms of lower-small-bowel obstruction are less severe, with less pain and shock, and include delayed and feculent vomiting. Obstruction in the upper jejunum diminishes urine output.

Pain in large-bowel obstruction is much less acute than in small-bowel blockage and shock is less frequent and severe, except with volvulus or intussusception. Distention is an early manifestation of large-bowel obstruction; vomiting occurs later. The length of time between bouts of pain can help locate the obstruction. A 4- to 5-minute period between attacks indicates small-bowel obstruction; a 10- to 15-minute period between attacks indicates large-bowel obstruction. During the third trimester, you can rule out early labor by auscultating and palpating the uterus during the bout of pain, as you may hear "rushes" of high-pitched bowel sounds.

Radiographically, air-fluid levels and distended loops of small bowel indicate small-bowel obstruction. "Hoop loops," transverse loops, "string-of-beads sign," and "coffee-bean sign" may also be seen. In large-bowel obstruction, the bowel is distended, with or without cecal distention, and air-fluid levels may be demonstrated. There may be secondary obstruction of the small bowel due to an incompetent ileocecal valve.

Intussusception during pregnancy is one of the most serious complications of bowel obstruction. Passage of a stool consisting of blood-streaked mucus—the "currant jelly" stool—is diagnostic. Uterine size may allow palpation of the sausage-shaped tumor.[16]

Midgut volvulus is secondary to a congenital defect either in the rotation of the midgut or in the attachment of the bowel to the posterior abdomen, or both. Torsion at the point of fixation, by the enlarging uterus, can cause partial obstruction and proximal distention. The decreased abdominal space prevents spontaneous detorsion. Sudden reduction in uterine size and a changed position of abdominal organs can also cause this problem. Barium enema seems to be the best way to identify it. Immediate surgery is mandatory, as bowel infarction is rapidly fatal.

To gain the best possible exposure and access to the bowel at operation, cesarean section may be necessary. However, it need not be done routinely.

Acute cholecystitis

Acute or chronic gallbladder disease is associated with gallstones in 85% to 95% of cases. Bile stasis, bacterial infection, or other factors account for the rest. The increased incidence of cholecystitis in pregnancy may be secondary to accelerated stone growth. There are three possible causes:

■ Increased progesterone slows gallbladder emptying.

■ A 50% increase in esterified and free blood cholesterol during pregnancy increases the amount of cholesterol in the bile.

■ Or the bile salt pool decreases.

Women taking exogenous estrogens in oral contraceptives or for postmenopausal replacement therapy are at a higher risk for gallstones, as are pregnant patients. The hormones affect cholesterol metabolism and smooth muscle tone of the gallbladder.

Acute and chronic symptoms seem to be the same for pregnant and nonpregnant patients. Right upper quadrant tenderness, the most frequent sign, is usually produced by cystic duct obstruction. Jaundice may accompany

43

common duct obstruction. The WBC is not of diagnostic value. The pain, described by the patient as lancing, colicky, or just a "deep ache," may be excruciating. It usually begins in the midepigastrium and radiates to the right upper quadrant around the sides to the back or directly to the scapula. Most patients describe a steady pain lasting 15 to 60 minutes. In nonpregnant patients, the gallbladder may be palpable, with a positive Murphy sign. The gallbladder can rarely be palpated in pregnancy. Nausea and vomiting or anorexia may accompany the onset of symptoms.

Oral cholecystogram and IV cholangiography, while helpful in nonpregnant patients, are contraindicated in pregnancy. Radiopaque calculi are most often seen, as is a soft tissue mass, but no clear-cut findings can be counted on. Sometimes there is a local ileus or basal chest change.

The postpartum period seems to be a time of greater susceptibility to gallstone attack than is gestation itself. Attacks during puerperium are generally more severe than during pregnancy.

Management is initially conservative, with intermittent nasogastric suctioning, administration of crystalloids IV, narcotics, and antibiotics if sepsis is evident or conservative therapy has produced no improvement after four days. Surgery is indicated for uncontrollable chronic disease or for an acute episode with peritonitis. The second trimester is best for surgery because the risk to the fetus is less and the uterus is not enlarged enough to encroach on the operative field. Surgery is more often necessary after delivery.

Peptic ulcer disease

We define peptic ulcer disease as the formation of ulcerations 1.0 mm to 1.0 cm or greater in diameter in the duodenal bulb, postbulbar area, distal antrum, and the pyloric channel of the upper GI tract. Pregnancy ameliorates peptic ulcer disease in two ways. Progesterone appears to lower gastric acid secretion and increase the production of gastric mucus. And histamine is inactivated or blocked by plasma histaminase, which is synthesized by the placenta and rises dramatically during pregnancy.

Attacks are characterized by moderate to severe burning, cramping, boring, or pressing pain. Discomfort lasts from 15 to 60 minutes, is relieved by food or antacid, and is exacerbated by ingestion of aspirin, coffee, or alcoholic beverages. Vomiting is rare unless an ulcer is present in the pyloric channel. Melena or hematemesis may be present secondary to erosion.

Complications arise from bleeding at the base of an ulcer, luminal obstruction secondary to edema or fibrosis in the region of the ulcer, or perforation into the peritoneal cavity or the pancreatic bed. Manage bleeding by endoscopy, nasogastric suction, cold isotonic saline lavage, and blood replacement.

Perforation is life-threatening and has a 100% mortality if treated by medical means alone. Symptoms of perforation can be divided into three stages.

1. **Prostration or primary shock.** There is great generalized abdominal pain, anxious and ashen appearance, subnormal temperature, small and weak pulse, shallow respirations, nausea and vomiting, and pain in one or both shoulders.

2. **Reaction or masked peritonitis.** The abdominal pain decreases, vomiting ceases, appearance improves, temperature is normal, pulse normal, respirations still shallow, abdominal wall very rigid and tender and/or flat. Movement induces pain.

3. **Frank peritonitis with toxic shock.** Vomiting becomes more frequent. The abdomen is distended and tender. The pulse is rapid and small, respirations labored and rapid, and the facial expression reflects pain and anxiety.

The diagnosis often can be made before frank peritonitis sets in and surgery becomes necessary. If complications develop late in the third trimester, cesarean section may be necessary to obtain better exposure and to protect the fetus from potential distress secondary to peritonitis and maternal hypotension.[17]

Radiographically, perforated peptic ulcer is best diagnosed by a finding of pneumoperitoneum. There may also be air-fluid levels, free fluid, and elevated diaphragms.

There is an increased frequency of peptic ulcer disease and exacerbation of symptoms and complications around the menopause. A differential diagnosis includes cholecystitis, acute pancreatitis, acute appendicitis, ischemic coronary artery disease, ischemic bowel disease, and stomach cancer.

Acute pancreatitis

In the nonpregnant patient, acute pancreatitis is usually associated with chronic alcoholism, gallstones, surgery, trauma, metabolic disorders, infections, drugs, connective tissue disease, penetrating duodenal ulcer, or obstruction of the ampulla of Vater. During pregnancy, the cause is usually gallstones (36%), infection (25%), toxemia (9%), chlorothiazides (8%), or alcohol consumption (1%). Stasis, increased concentration of cholesterol in bile, and changes in the physicochemical nature of bile salts—all factors believed important in the formation of biliary calculi—occur in normal pregnancy. Pancreatitis commonly occurs in conjunction with or secondary to gallbladder disease. Lymphatic transmission of inflammatory disease within the pancreaticobiliary system may be involved.

Initially, inflammation of the pancreas liberates proteolytic enzymes that begin to digest pancreatic and peripancreatic tissues. This process liberates other active enzymes, continuing the process of autodigestion. Necrotizing pancreatitis develops. It may resolve with medical management or may continue, with associated symptoms of systemic deterioration, including circulatory collapse, renal and respiratory failure, and hypocalcemia. While calcium levels normally are somewhat depressed during pregnancy, hypocalcemia accompanying severe pancreatitis is a poor prognostic sign. Death has occurred in most patients whose serum calcium levels fell below 7.0 mg%.[18]

Fever without other complications is unusual and the WBC is generally not helpful. The incidence of proteinuria is very high. Blood electrolyte derangements reflect the severity of vomiting. Liver function tests will be abnormal when there is concomitant biliary-tract disease.

Epigastric pain and guarding may be significant but the diagnosis is made by confirming an elevation of the serum amylase and diastase (urinary amylase). Serum amylase levels peak 6 to 12 hours after the onset of symptoms and return to normal within 24 to 72 hours. However, the diastase levels remain elevated for seven to 10 days.

Radiographically, the most reliable x-ray finding is the "sentinel-loop sign," in which one or more loops of jejunum are seen in the left upper quadrant of the abdomen. There may also be a localized ileus of the stomach or duodenum. Another occasional finding is the "colon cut-off sign" where the large bowel is dilated in either the hepatic or splenic flexure. Pleural effusion, left greater than right, has also been reported.

Management centers on putting the pancreas to rest: nothing taken orally, intermittent nasogastric suction, analgesics—meperidine hydrochloride (Demerol) is the drug of choice, IV fluids, and antiemetics. Anticholinergics, glucagon, and antibiotics do not appear to be of therapeutic benefit.

Most complications are associated with the severe necrotizing or hemorrhagic type of pancreatitis, and are secondary to local inflammation and the necrotic effects of pancreatic enzymes on peripancreatic tissues, or a remote effect of circulating enzymes. Laparotomy is indicated only when the diagnosis is not definite or toxic pancreatic exudate must be removed with a wide sump drain. There is no reason to terminate pregnancy, as there is no proof that pregnancy adversely affects the prognosis.

The differential diagnosis in women of childbearing age includes perforated viscus, especially from peptic ulcer, cholecystitis, acute intestinal obstruction, renal disease, dissecting aortic aneurysm, pneumonia, and diabetic ketoacidosis.

REFERENCES

1. Saunders P, Milton PJD: Laparotomy during pregnancy: An assessment of diagnostic accuracy and fetal wastage. Br Med J 13:165, 1973
2. Devore GR: Acute abdominal pain in the pregnant patient due to pancreatitis, acute appendicitis, cholecystitis, or peptic ulcer disease. Clin Perinatol 7:349, 1980
3. Farquharson RG: Acute appendicitis in pregnancy. Scott Med J 25:36, 1980
4. Lee PWR: The plain x-ray in the acute abdomen: A surgeon's evaluation. Br J Surg 63:763, 1976
5. Gilstrap LC, Cunningham FG, Whalley PG: Acute pyelonephritis in pregnancy: An anterospective study. Obstet Gynecol 57:409, 1981
6. Cope A: *The Early Diagnosis of the Acute Abdomen:* New York: Oxford University Press, 1972
7. Munro A, Jones PF: Abdominal emergencies in the puerperium. Br Med J 691: 1975
8. Stern JL, Buscema J, Rosensheim NB, et al: Spontaneous rupture of benign cystic teratomas. Obstet Gynecol 57:363, 1981
9. Hamlin E Jr, Bartlett MD, Smith JA: Acute surgical emergencies of the abdomen in pregnancy. N Engl J Med 244:128, 1951
10. Anderson GV, Bucklew WB: Abdominal surgery and tubo-ovarian abscesses. West J Surg Obstet Gynecol 70:67, 1962
11. Nebel WA, Lucas WE: Management of tubo-ovarian abscess in pregnancy. Obstet Gynecol 32:382, 1968
12. Hunt SM, Kimchloe BW, Schriver PC: Tubo-ovarian abscess in pregnancy. Obstet Gynecol 43:57, 1974
13. Hill LM, Symmonds RE: Small bowel obstruction in pregnancy. Obstet Gynecol 49:170, 1977
14. Milne B, Johnstone MS: Intestinal obstruction in pregnancy. Scott Med J 24:80 1979
15. Crouch M: The acute abdomen in women. Practitioner 222:457, 1979
16. Svesko VS, Pisani BJ: Intestinal obstruction in pregnancy. Am J Obstet Gynecol 71:157, 1960
17. Becker-Anderson H, Husfeldt V: Peptic ulcer in pregnancy. Acta Obstet Gynecol Scand 50:371, 1971
18. Corlett RC, Mishell DR: Pancreatitis in pregnancy. Am J Obstet Gynecol 113:281, 1972

How good is emergency training for ob/gyn residents?

Some experts believe most of today's programs afford residents sufficient expertise and experience, while others find only a few programs adequate. Everyone has ideas about how the training should be done.

Many institutions now realize the importance of teaching house staff emergency procedures and providing experience in using them. According to Hervy E. Averette, MD, Professor and Director, Division of Gynecologic Oncology, at the University of Miami School of Medicine, even programs that are not entirely adequate in every respect offer cardiopulmonary resuscitation (CPR) to all physicians, even attendings. In fact, completing an approved course is a necessary requirement for certification.

However, even CPR training may not always be as thorough as might be wished. In a letter in the *New England Journal of Medicine* [303:1534, 1980], Marc Nelson, MS, points out that while any physician can grasp the theory in minutes, mastering correct technique may require from 8 to 10 hours. "Merely being a doctor does not speed up this process any more than it would facilitate learning how to ride a bicycle," he writes. Another letter in the same issue, from M. Clagett Collins, MD, and John M. Packard, MD, proposes that the Joint Commission on Accreditation of Hospitals require that all physicians who work in critical-care settings be certified in advanced cardiac life support.

And Joseph Collea, MD, Director of Residency Training at Georgetown University

School of Medicine, Washington, D.C., thinks an advanced course is essential for all residents. If a patient suffers a cardiac or respiratory arrest on the operating table, he says, "you need to know what to do until the cardiac-arrest team arrives. In such emergencies, the anesthesiologist is there to provide ventilation, but the surgeon needs to know what drugs to use and how to use them, and how to read the ECG."

Advanced CPR training is only the beginning, says *Contemporary Ob/Gyn* Editor-in-Chief John T. Queenan, MD, Professor and Chairman, Department of Obstetrics and Gynecology, Georgetown University School of Medicine. He believes a rotation through anesthesiology is basic, because "that's what teaches people how to handle emergencies." Any normal procedure may suddenly turn into an emergency, notes Queenan. "Physicians must be able to respond well to the unexpected emergency—a cardiac arrest, amniotic fluid embolus, postpartum hemorrhage."

"The difference between a well-trained obstetrician and a midwife," Queenan believes, "is that the doctor can handle the unexpected, while the midwife has been trained mainly to handle the routine. Being able to function well in an emergency is an extension of being able to handle the unexpected."

"Residents see gynecologic and obstetric emergencies every day of the week at LAC/USC Medical Center, where I trained," says Thomas J. Benedetti, MD, Assistant Professor of Obstetrics and Gynecology, University of Washington School of Medicine, Seattle. "We ob/gyn residents ran our own emergency room," he says, adding that in institutions where this is not the case, someone else may do the initial workup and the resident in ob-gyn may be called after the fact. "In such situations, their hands-on experience could be fairly limited," Benedetti continues. "Where I am now, our emergency room is staffed by emergency room physicians, but most gynecologic patients are seen immediately by a resident in gynecology. After residency, you don't deal with as many emergencies. Skills may atrophy unless they are used regularly. Frequent retraining is essential if emergency medicine skills are to be maintained."

Are specialists in ER the answer?

Some experts believe that only physicians who see emergencies on a regular basis are competent to handle them. According to Gail

V. Anderson, MD, Director of Emergency, LAC-USC Medical Center, and Chairman and Professor, Department of Emergency Medicine, University of Southern California School of Medicine, Los Angeles, "Many if not most specialists think they are competent in emergencies within their area, but it's not true. Unfortunately, they don't find that out until they get into a life-threatening situation." It was to fill this need that the specialty of emergency medicine was established, he says.

Anderson was the first professor and chairman of emergency medicine in the U.S. For 10 years, he was Professor and Chairman of the Department of Obstetrics and Gynecology at LAC/USC, where he dealt almost entirely with acute aspects of the specialty—septic shock, ruptured tubo-ovarian abscess, infection in pregnancy, diabetic pregnancy, ruptured uteri in grand multiparas.

The problem, as he perceived it, was that residents who went into private practice and stopped seeing emergencies on a regular basis lost many of the skills they had acquired during the residency. The solution, Anderson concluded, was to train some physicians to do only emergency medicine. The American College of Emergency Physicians was chartered in 1968, and the American Board of Emergency Medicine in 1976. There are now 248 physicians certified by the ABEM. "Another thousand will be certified in 1981," Anderson says, and he reports there are now 35 to 40 training programs, for a total of about 400 residency positions in emergency medicine.

Training programs are necessary for those wishing to specialize in emergency medicine, Anderson says, because "the training the ob/gyn resident gets in the usual program in handling emergencies is minimal." But he finds "a lot of resistance to the idea, particularly in the Northeast. It is not catching on as it has in the Midwest and West."

Georgetown's Collea disagrees that all life-threatening situations should be left to one ER physician. He points out that, years ago, most physicians were generalists. Later, "we thought everybody had to be superspecialized. Now we have the ER specialist, who treats everybody. With that," he says, "we've come full circle." Collea thinks it's impossible to train one physician to treat every emergency, from a foreign body in the ear to a bleeding ulcer. "That's why we have specialists," he says.

His opinion is seconded by Gerard W. Ostheimer, MD, Assistant Professor of Anesthesia, Harvard Medical School, and Associate Director of Obstetric Anesthesia, Brigham and Women's Hospital, Boston: "Most physicians who are not obstetrician-gynecologists are unable to respond to the special needs of women patients, and that generalization applies equally to emergency situations."

"In our ER, residents are the first line of defense, and the system works well," says Ostheimer. The ER is staffed by an intern or two in each general specialty—surgery or medicine—and a resident in each specialty, including ob/gyn, is available immediately. ER care, Ostheimer believes, is an integral part of every resident's education.

More than once, Ostheimer says, he's seen physicians specially trained in emergency medicine "drop the ball." They see a woman complaining of some vaginal bleeding, forget the possibility she may be pregnant, and do an incautious examination. This may start the patient bleeding in earnest—if, for example, the examiner penetrates a central placenta previa. The specialist in ob/gyn would suspect placenta previa and understand that a pelvic exam might induce hemorrhage.

Another typically mismanaged case is that of the woman who reports a small amount of lower abdominal discomfort. She is tentatively diagnosed as having some unidentified gastrointestinal problem and tests are ordered. Two days later, she's in borderline shock because the ER physician failed to recognize chronic ectopic pregnancy.

"The ER physicians don't know enough about women's problems," Ostheimer concludes. "They're fine for cardiacs and accidents, but they lack expertise in ob/gyn." However, Anderson thinks ER physicians can and should be trained to recognize and treat these problems, because an ob/gyn specialist is not always immediately available.

What's the best way?

While Ostheimer recommends a special room within the ER for ob/gyn patients, to which residents are summoned (by the admitting ER nurse) when needed, Averette believes residents should rotate through the critical-care unit. "That's the only way they can learn what they can do and what their limitations are," he says.

He cites the case of patients with pre-eclampsia. These patients' problems are different, physiologically, from those of patients with crushed chests. He thinks it's essential that the admitting physician be the one who continues to care for the patient.

Collea agrees with LAC/USC's Anderson that an ER program is needed to train residents to recognize a wide range of problems, but prefers to see each specialist trained in ER procedures for that specialty. Collea cites his own experience at Johns Hopkins, where "an ambulance pulled up every few minutes. A triage officer, a senior resident, made a quick decision and sent the patient to the correct specialist. We treated a wide range of problems—active bleeding, acute PID, and ectopics, among others."

Years ago, according to Collea, a resident in a small community-hospital program was able to learn the basics because "there wasn't that much to know. With our explosion of information today, however, residents must be exposed to many more patients."

"Smaller is a relative term," says Philip B. Mead, MD, Professor and Director of Residency Training, Department of Obstetrics and Gynecology, University of Vermont College of Medicine, Burlington. "Our emergencies are exactly the same as those at the huge centers," he says. "The numbers are lower, but percentage-wise we see as many cases." Mead thinks the important question is: Where does your hospital fit into the total health-care picture? He points out that to give each resident equivalent experience, a program with 48 residents must manage four times as many emergencies as a program with 12 residents.

Physicians in large cities don't really understand the rural situation, Mead contends. "They know that a small private hospital near a huge center sees few patients with acute emergencies, because they go to the center. But ours is the only hospital in a large area and we see everything."

His opinion is seconded by S. Ender Dolen, MD, Assistant Professor of Obstetrics and Gynecology at Texas Tech University Health Science Center, and Director of the Residency Program at Lubbock General Hospital. "I saw fewer emergencies at the State University of New York at Buffalo, where I was one of 40 residents, than our residents see here. All the emergencies within a 250-mile radius come to us," he says. The triage officer is a specialist in emergency medicine, soon to be board certified, Dolen says. He summons a resident in ob/gyn to see all the ob/gyn emergencies.

Residents at the University of Vermont spend two months in the ER, where they see all kinds of patients. They spend a month in the intensive-care nursery and a month in the adult special-care unit, learning how to manage critically ill patients. They also rotate through the oncology service.

"We have a very active oncology program, but no oncology fellows," Mead says. He points out that many of the seriously ill patients in ob/gyn are on the oncology services. When there are oncology fellows, the residents in ob/gyn don't feel the same primary responsibility for managing patients in pulmonary edema, in septic shock, or patients who "blow out their femoral arteries after a groin dissection."

Says Mead, "When the fat's in the fire, most residents call the oncology fellows. In programs such as ours, where the ob/gyn residents participate actively and primarily in the oncology service, they're capable of dealing with acute emergencies themselves. Even our first-year residents learn to put in subclavian lines routinely."

Mead stresses that size alone is a poor criterion of a good program. However, he agrees with Collea that inadequate programs must be phased out. This process has already begun, Collea says. The Council on Resident Education in Obstetrics and Gynecology (CREOG) establishes what basic materials residents are expected to learn. Then, if residency review committees find that a program doesn't fulfill the criteria, it's not approved and its residents are not permitted to take their boards.

Denis Cavanagh, MD
Robert A. Knuppel, MD, MPH

Treatment priorities for the ob patient in shock

First, give oxygen by mask or respirator. Then, replace intravascular fluid volume. In general, turn to drug or surgical treatment of the hemorrhage only after ventilation and infusion are assured.

Hemorrhagic shock is the most frequent cause of maternal death in the U.S. (Table 7-1). Severe blood loss may result from ruptured ectopic pregnancy, abortion, ruptured uterus, placenta previa, abruptio placentae, or postpartum hemorrhage.[1] Prompt and adequate filling of the intravascular space is necessary to preserve life. The patient's vital signs may be misleading in assessing the effect of blood loss; for example, a normal or even slightly elevated blood pressure does not preclude life-threatening hypovolemia, nor do low pulse rates.

Pathophysiology

When blood is lost from the vascular space and the circulating blood volume is diminished, the catecholamine level rises and the arterioles and veins constrict. The liberation of pressor substances helps sustain this vasoconstriction, and renal blood flow is redistributed within the kidney to protect the medulla. Flow to the splanchnic, uterine, renal, muscular, and cutaneous organs decreases, whereas flow to the brain and heart increases. In this early phase, which is compensated and reversible, extravascular fluid flows into the

Table 7-1. Causes of maternal mortality in U.S.*

Cause	1975	1976	1977	1978	Total
Hemorrhage†	125	110	120	89	408
Sepsis	76	71	70	61	278
Eclamptogenic toxemia	77	83	55	62	277
All other	125	126	128	107	486
Total	403	390	373	319	1,449

*National Center for Health Statistics.[10-12]
†Ruptured ectopic pregnancy, abortion, ruptured uterus, placenta previa, abruptio placentae, and postpartum.

vascular compartment. Venous return and cardiac output are maintained, as the circulating volume accommodates itself to the vascular space. Tachycardia also helps maintain cardiac output. Provided bleeding is controlled, IV fluids and electrolytes readily achieve homeostasis.

If the hemorrhagic process continues, however, arteriolar and capillary tone is lost, and the capillary bed and vascular compartment expand. Metabolic acidosis, at times associated with disseminated intravascular coagulation (DIC) and stimulation of the fibrinolytic system, marks this secondary stage of late decompensation. Hepatic, renal, cardiopulmonary, or CNS failure signals the transition to irreversible hemorrhagic shock.

Clinical picture

Shock has a reversible, primary stage with an early (warm) or compensated phase and a late (cold) or decompensated phase; then, if unchecked, it progresses to an irreversible secondary stage. The signs and expected response to volume replacement of each stage are outlined in Table 7-2. In the early phase, there is relatively normal blood pressure, tachycardia, and diaphoresis. The patient appears restless and anxious. You can manage this compensated phase easily by volume replacement.

If you don't treat early, the hypotensive phase follows. At the beginning, you can readily control this phase with adequate volume replacement. As the process evolves, treatment elicits a much less satisfactory response. Even when you intensify treatment, the patient may still enter the secondary or irreversible stage. However, you can often reverse hemorrhagic shock very late in its

Table 7-2. Evolution of hemorrhagic shock and expected response to volume replacement*

	Primary shock		Secondary shock
	Early	**Late**	
Clinical picture:			
Mental state	Alert and anxious	Confused	Coma
General appearance	Normal and warm	Pale and cold	Cyanotic and cold
Blood pressure	Slightly hypotensive	Moderately hypotensive	Markedly hypotensive
Respiratory system	Slight tachypnea	Tachypnea	Tachypnea (and cyanosis)
Urinary output	30–60 ml/hr	30 ml/hr	Anuria
Effect of volume challenge:			
Blood pressure	Increased	Slightly increased	No response
Urinary output	Increased	Slightly increased	No response

*Cavanagh D, Knuppel RA.[13]

evolution. For this reason, begin vigorous therapy as soon as you diagnose shock, even when the patient appears exsanguinated.

General plan of action for combating shock

It is important to do the therapeutic and diagnostic maneuvers in proper sequence.[2] The approach shown in Table 7-3 is more valuable than such time-honored routines as prolonged head-down position, which only makes breathing more difficult for an already hypoxic patient.

Ventilation. The most frequent cause of death in shock patients is inadequate respiratory exchange. Measure pH, partial pressure of

Table 7-3. Therapeutic steps in treating hemorrhagic shock*

Priority	Therapy	Purpose
1	Ventilation	Provide adequate pulmonary CO_2 and O_2 exchange
2	Infusion	Maintain blood volume with fluid and electrolyte balance
3	Pump restoration	Restore cardiac competence
4	Pharmacologic	Improve perfusion by vasoactive agents
5	Specific	Treat primary causes medically and surgically

*Cavanagh D, Knuppel RA.[13]

oxygen (Po_2), and partial pressure of carbon dioxide (Pco_2) in arterial blood. The patient has respiratory acidosis when the Po_2 in arterial blood is less than 70 mm Hg, the Pco_2 more than 45 mm Hg, and the pH less than 7.35. Try to return the arterial Po_2 to normal as soon as possible to reduce tissue hypoxia.

Infusion. Combat shock with adequate blood volume, colloids (5% serum albumin), or crystalloids. Use the central venous pressure (CVP), the pulmonary artery wedge pressure (PAWP), the blood volume estimation, and the urinary output as guides to the fluid intake requirements. You can assess cardiac competence in a patient with borderline CVP (12 to 16 cm H_2O) by infusing 500 ml of fluid at a rate of 20 ml/minute. If the CVP rises no more than 5 cm H_2O and returns to within 2 cm of the initial level, the myocardium is competent. The pump must be effective; therefore maintain or restore cardiac competence to achieve adequate circulating blood volume.

Pharmacologic and surgical treatment. Administer drugs to combat shock only after you have given oxygen and replaced fluids. When there is massive intra-abdominal hemorrhage, however, you may have to operate immediately to stop the bleeding.

Monitoring the patient. Unless you have definite evidence of intra-abdominal bleeding, as in ectopic pregnancy or uterine rupture, defer surgery until other measures to control shock have been taken. In postpartum hemorrhage, give oxytocin for uterine atony or repair a cervical laceration without delay.

Prostaglandins have recently been used to control postpartum hemorrhage. Systemic administration, by continuous IV infusion or by gluteal IM injection, does not achieve complete hemostasis, but local administration, by direct injection into the uterine musculature transabdominally or transvaginally, dramatically reduces the rate of bleeding.[3] Investigations are under way to evaluate other forms of prostaglandins for control of uterine atony.[4]

Transfusion therapy. As you restore hemostasis, you must watch for DIC or dilution of clotting factors. The indications for whole blood have decreased as more versatile and economical preparations of red blood cell concentrates have become available. However, if whole blood less than six days old is available, clotting factors will not be a concern.

Patients with chronic anemias often have expanded plasma volumes and risk congestive heart failure if whole blood is transfused. The initial transfusion rate should not exceed 100 ml/hour. Watch the patient carefully. Losses up to 1,000 ml usually can be corrected by a colloidal or salt solution. During a massive transfusion, the plasma coagulation factors and platelets will be diluted and not adequately replaced by stored blood. All coagulation factors except factor VIII may be supplied by transfusion of whole blood less than seven days old (Table 7-4).

A preferable alternative would be to transfuse a unit of fresh frozen plasma for every five units of packed red cells.[5] The platelet count falls in proportion to the number of units transfused; with transfusions of more than 15 units, the platelet count will usually fall below 100,000/cu mm. If bleeding contin-

Table 7-4. Blood replacement therapy for obstetric coagulation failure*

Component	Unit volume (ml)	Factors present
Fresh whole blood	500	All, including platelets
Fresh-frozen plasma	200 or 400	All, except platelets
Fresh-dried plasma	400	All, except platelets
Platelet-rich plasma	200	All, and viable platelets
Platelet concentrates	35–50	Viable platelets
Cryoprecipitate	20–50	Fibrinogen, VIII, and XIII
Fibrinogen	200–300	Fibrinogen (1–2 gm)

*Cavanagh D, Knuppel RA.[13]

ues because of thrombocytopenia, transfuse platelets.

Medical management. Give oxygen by mask or respirator at 6 to 8 liters/minute. Make sure the airway is adequate. Replace intravascular fluid volume, and whenever possible replace blood with blood. Always use a large-bore needle (18 gauge), or indwelling polyethylene catheter (16 gauge), to ensure rapid replacement. For early hemorrhagic shock, give IV fluids and electrolytes.

More severe hemorrhagic shock demands properly typed and cross-matched blood. For severe hemorrnage, the blood should be as fresh as possible, and in quantities sufficient to replace the estimated loss or until all clinical evidence of shock has subsided. When blood is unavailable, give serum albumin, dextran, or 3% saline.

Arterial blood pressure is a poor guide to the management of hemorrhage in obstetric patients, because they are well able to compensate for blood loss. This is particularly so in abruptio placentae; therefore, use CVP or PAWP as guides.[6-8] Early and adequate replacement is especially difficult to achieve in abruption, because of the tendency to underestimate blood loss.

Use vasopressors as little as possible because shock escalates peripheral vasoconstriction. To combat acidosis, use 5% dextrose in normal saline, with sodium bicarbonate added. Ringer's lactate solution is less suitable for patients in shock, who are producing large amounts of lactate by the process of anaerobic metabolism.

Surgical management. Once you've instituted medical measures to combat shock, operate to attain hemostasis. The magnitude of the surgery will depend on the underlying condition. Although it is usually preferable to defer surgery until the patient is out of shock, sometimes, as in severe hemorrhage from rupture of the gravid uterus, it is impractical to wait for responses to medical measures. When a blood-filled abdomen is opened, manual compression of the aorta against the vertebral column and removal of clots will often allow better visualization of the bleeding site.

Identifiable bleeding points can be controlled with proper suturing. Rupture of the gravid uterus usually calls for total abdominal hysterectomy. In rare cases, if the defect is small, you may try to repair it. However, there is always the hazard of another rupture with a subsequent pregnancy.

Ligation of the hypogastric arteries is often useful. If bleeding is from the uterus, ligate the ovarian vessels bilaterally before ligating the hypogastric arteries. Make sure you have identified the ureter; usually this is easiest to do where it crosses the common iliac artery. Proceed as follows: Isolate the bifurcation of the iliac arteries, identify the internal iliac artery, and double ligate its anterior division, with #0 silk suture, close to its origin. This procedure has few adverse effects. If possible, tie both hypogastric arteries. Do not transect them. Take care not to damage the hypogastric vein, because bleeding will be troublesome and difficult to control. Embolization of the hypogastric arteries to control vaginal bleeding has been suggested.[9] This technique is not without risk and further experience will be necessary before its true value is established.

In the interest of educating residents we frequently perform a "sham" bilateral hypogastric ligation, because the procedure is rarely indicated clinically. This sham operation affords residents an opportunity to learn the technique, and protects patients who need the operation from dangerous attempts by the untutored "occasional" operator.

REFERENCES

1. Cavanagh D, Knuppel RA, Copeland WJ, et al: Hemorrhagic shock in the obstetric patient. In Sakamoto S, Tojo S, Nakayama T (eds): *International Congress Series 512 Proceedings of the IX World Congress of Gynecology & Obstetrics, Tokyo, Aclata 25-31, 1979.* Princeton, N.J.: Excerpta Medica, 1979
2. Weil MH, Shubin H (eds): *Critical Care Medicine.* Hagerstown, Md.: Harper & Row, 1976
3. Takagi T, Yoshida T, Togo Y, et al: The effects of intramyometrial injection of prostaglandin $F_{2\alpha}$ on severe postpartum hemorrhage. Prostaglandins 12:565, 1976
4. Hayashi R: Personal communication, 1981
5. Cooksey JA, Orlina AR: Blood and blood products replacement therapy. J Reprod Med 19:233, 1977
6. O'Driscoll K, McCarthy JR: J Obstet Gynaecol Br Commonw 73:923, 1966
7. Swan JJG, Ganz W, Forrester J, et al: N Engl J Med 284:447, 1970
8. Cotton DB, Benedetti TJ: Use of the Swan-Ganz catheter in obstetrics and gynecology. Obstet Gynecol 56:641, 1980
9. Smith DC, Wyatt JF: Embolization of the hypogastric arteries in the control of massive vaginal hemorrhage. Obstet Gynecol 49:317, 1977
10. National Center for Health Statistics, Department of Health, Education and Welfare: Vital Health Stat 30:11, 1975
11. National Center for Health Statistics, Department of Health, Education and Welfare: Vital Health Stat 26:12, 1976
12. National Center for Health Statistics, Department of Health, Education and Welfare: Vital Health Stat 28:1, 1977
13. Cavanagh D, Knuppel RA: *Obstetric Emergencies,* ed 3. New York: Harper & Row, 1981

Gregory C. Bolton, MD
Fredric L. Cohen, MD

Detecting and treating ectopic pregnancy

The incidence of extrauterine pregnancy has almost doubled in the past 10 years. It accounts for 10% of all maternal deaths.

Early diagnosis and aggressive surgical management can save as many as 75% of these patients.

The leading cause of maternal mortality during the first trimester of pregnancy, ectopic pregnancy remains very difficult to diagnose. This is primarily because it is relatively asymptomatic in the early weeks of pregnancy. The onset of symptoms often heralds acute rupture and sudden massive hemorrhage. Early diagnosis, aggressive surgical management, and adequate blood and fluid replacement could save 75% of these patients, most of whom have visited a physician days before the actual rupture.

The overall incidence of extrauterine implantation of the fertilized ovum (blastocyst) in the U.S. is from 1:84 to 1:230—approximately 1% of all deliveries. In the past decade alone, while the annual number of maternal deaths decreased, the number of ectopic pregnancies increased from 15,000 to 40,000 a year. The increase is attributable to the rising incidence of sexually transmitted disease that corresponds with more sex partners, and the double-edged sword of modern antibiotic therapy. The proportion of all maternal deaths secondary to ectopic pregnancies is now 10%. (In nonwhite patients, ectopic pregnancy has become the single largest cause of maternal death.)

Major sites of extrauterine implantation include all segments of the fallopian tube (90%), the ovary (0.1%), uterine cornua (0.6%), cervix (0.1%), and peritoneal cavity (1.3%) (Figure 8-1). Most tubal gestations occur in the ampullary and isthmic portions of the tube.

What causes extrauterine pregnancy?

Partial occlusion of the fallopian tube allows conception to occur but often prevents passage of the fertilized egg into the uterine cavity. The success of current antibiotics in treating pelvic inflammatory disease often prevents total tubal occlusion. Occlusion tends to be more common in nongonococcal than in gonococcal salpingitis, probably because of the gonococcus's greater sensitivity to a wide variety of antibiotics. Following an infectious insult, the tubal lumen forms synechial bands that, along with agglutination of the tubal cilia, result in varying degrees of occlusion. One prospective study showed histologic evidence of chronic salpingitis in 50% to 55% of patients who have had infections. The likelihood of tubal occlusion increases with each subsequent infection: 12% with the first infection, 30% with the second infection, and 75% with the third episode.

The widespread use of IUDs also seems to have influenced the rate of extrauterine pregnancy. This association was first recognized by Grafenberg in 1929. A summary of the published literature on ectopic pregnancy, by Tatum and Schmidt, revealed that 1:23 or 4.3% of pregnancies occurring with an IUD in place were ectopic. The IUD seems to reduce uterine implantation of the ovum far more effectively than it reduces either tubal or ovarian implantation. In short, it does not protect against ectopic implantation in predisposed patients. IUD users also seem to be at greater risk immediately after the IUD is removed, and pregnancy should therefore be avoided for approximately two to three months after removal. The 1980 Women's Health Study Collaborative drew the following conclusions on the relationship between IUDs and ectopic pregnancy:

■ In the aggregate, women who have used an IUD in the past but are not using it now have the same risk of ectopic pregnancy as women who have never used one.

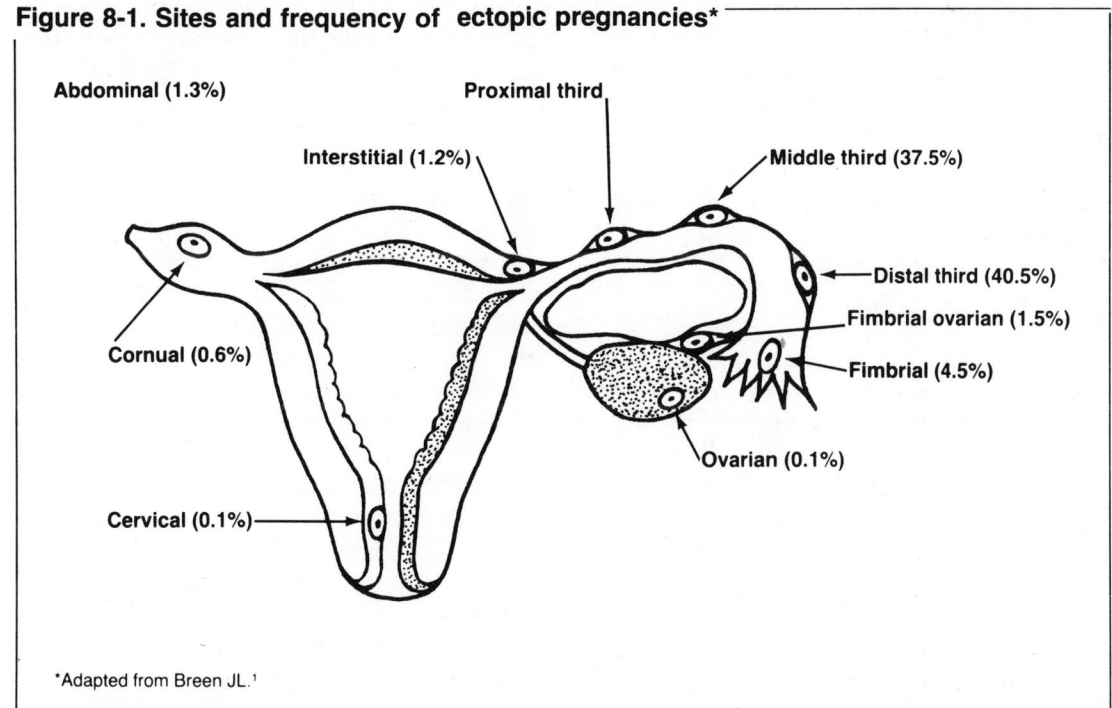

Figure 8-1. Sites and frequency of ectopic pregnancies*

- Abdominal (1.3%)
- Interstitial (1.2%)
- Proximal third
- Middle third (37.5%)
- Distal third (40.5%)
- Fimbrial ovarian (1.5%)
- Fimbrial (4.5%)
- Cornual (0.6%)
- Ovarian (0.1%)
- Cervical (0.1%)

*Adapted from Breen JL.[1]

- Current use of any form of contraception, including the IUD, decreases one's risk of ectopic pregnancy.
- IUD users have three times the risk of ectopic pregnancy that oral contraceptive users have and a risk equal to that of barrier contraceptive users.

Progesterone-only OCs increase the risk of ectopic pregnancy. This is thought to be secondary to minimal propulsive effects on the oviduct at the ampullary-isthmic junction and increasing incidence of ovum trapping.

Finally, our increased ability to restore tubal patency surgically increases the incidence. Women who have had such repair are at high risk of ectopic pregnancy. The common denominator in extrauterine pregnancy is delay of fertilized ovum transport from the site of ovulation to the uterine cavity.

Making the diagnosis

Accurate diagnosis and prompt management depend on clinical suspicion and careful assessment of symptoms and physical findings. Essentially, any woman—regardless of childbearing age or method of birth control, including tubal ligation—who complains of an irregular bleeding pattern and pain, needs evaluation for ectopic pregnancy. The classic triad of pain, bleeding, and adnexal mass is present in 75% of cases, but this figure varies according to how willing the patient in pain may be to let you examine her, the diagnostic skill of the examiner, and the duration of the pregnancy. Pain is almost always the most important feature and the symptom that first causes the patient to seek medical attention. Bleeding patterns and menstrual history vary from normal to highly irregular. Some form of bleeding takes place around the time of the expected menses in 50% of patients and about 50% of women have a five- to 10-week period of amenorrhea before other clinical signs appear. Over 50% of patients have "normal menses" four to eight weeks before admission and up to 20% have no history of a missed period. Pain is present for less than 24 hours in 45% of cases, from one to seven days in 30%, and more than one week in 25%. The location of the pain varies; there is adnexal tenderness in 95% of patients, bilateral tenderness in 43%, and pain on the side opposite the ectopic in 20% (Figure 8-2).

Pregnancy testing is of doubtful diagnostic value. Radioimmunoassay and radioreceptor assay have increased our accuracy in detecting an early pregnancy, but they can't identify its location.

Ultrasonic examination is helpful if the technique is performed correctly. An intrauterine gestational sac can be located consistently after five weeks' gestation. The presence of an intact sac should preclude suspicion of ectopic pregnancy, although dual pregnancy—intrauterine and ectopic—has been reported.

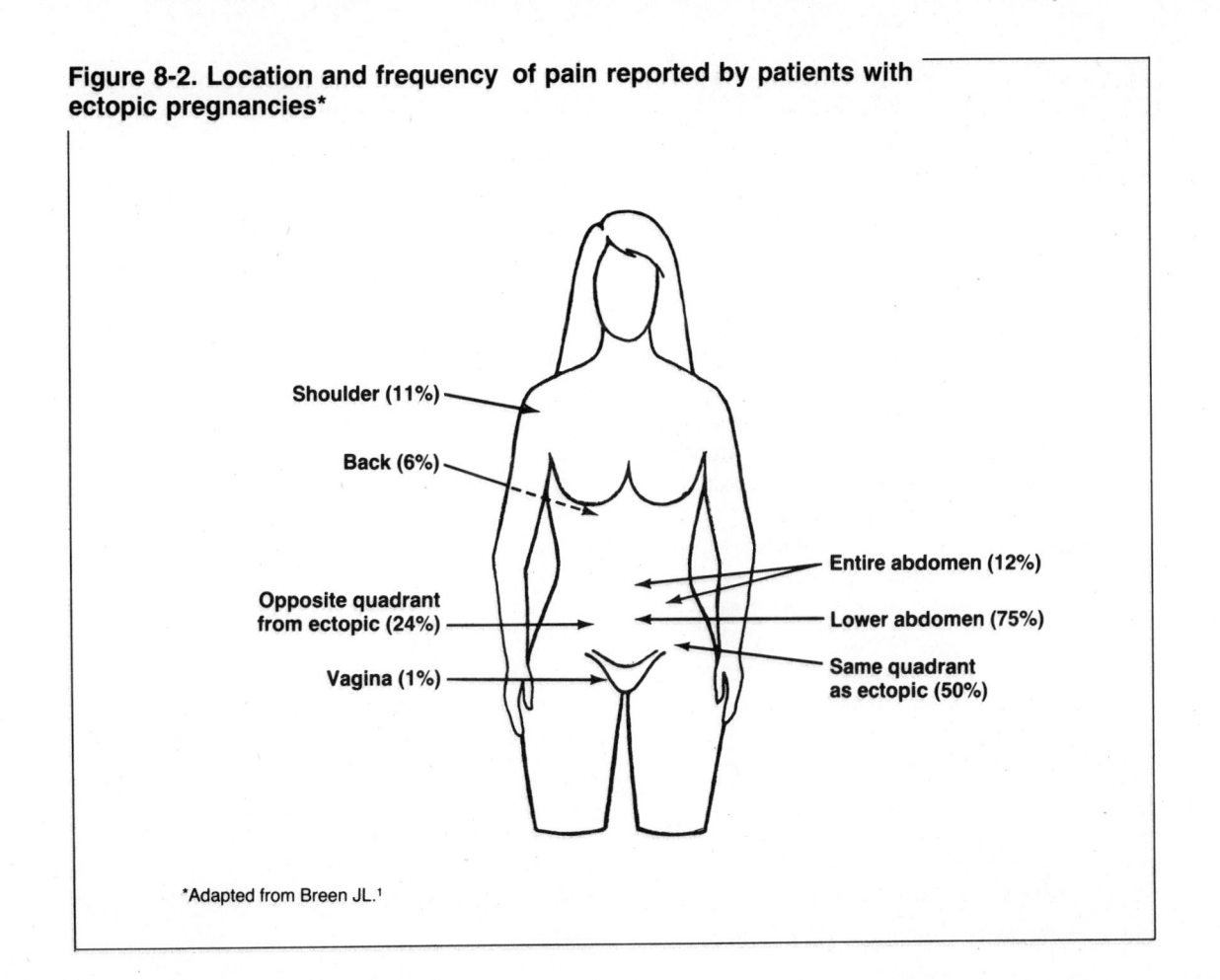

Figure 8-2. Location and frequency of pain reported by patients with ectopic pregnancies*

- Shoulder (11%)
- Back (6%)
- Entire abdomen (12%)
- Opposite quadrant from ectopic (24%)
- Lower abdomen (75%)
- Vagina (1%)
- Same quadrant as ectopic (50%)

*Adapted from Breen JL.[1]

Culdocentesis is helpful if ultrasound is not available, and it is a quick, easy way to identify intraperitoneal bleeding before hospital admission. The simple procedure of inserting a spinal needle attached to an aspirating syringe into the cul-de-sac between the uterosacral ligaments can be carried out in almost any situation when the diagnosis is in doubt.

If the patient does not desire to keep an intrauterine pregnancy, D & C can be useful for evaluating endometrial tissue. The presence of decidua and the absence of chorionic villi, along with pain and an adnexal mass, mandate visual inspection of the adnexa before an ectopic pregnancy can be ruled out.

Diagnostic laparoscopy is probably the major improvement in our ability to diagnose pelvic disease within the past decade. Its use is essential, except when precluded by hemodynamic instability; emergency laparotomy is indicated in such cases. Laparoscopy has replaced the more difficult and cumbersome technique of culdoscopy and often saves patients an unnecessary exploratory laparotomy. A laparotomy is still mandatory in the presence of hemoperitonium when culdocentesis is positive and diagnostic laparoscopy inadequate, so that the source and extent of the bleeding cannot be accurately defined.

Surgical approaches

The primary treatment for ectopic pregnancy remains surgical. The clinician must consider the location of the ectopic pregnancy, the patient's hemodynamic stability, and her desire for more children. Salpingectomy, the classic treatment for removal of ectopic pregnancy, is still the procedure of choice in most cases. Salpingectomy obviates any chance of recurrence, especially in conjunction with ipsilateral cornual resection. However, when fimbrial ectopic pregnancy or distal tubal abortion is found, a tubal extraction or "milking" procedure may evacuate the ectopic products without disrupting the integrity of the tube. If you can accomplish this easily without damaging tubal structure, while achieving adequate hemostasis, you may be able to preserve tubal function. When the pregnancy occurs in the patient's remaining tube, or when the contralateral tube is obviously seriously compromised from pre-existing disease, you may wish to consider a conservative approach to removing the fetus.

In experienced hands, salpingostomy—linear exposure of the unruptured ectopic sac—with removal and subsequent restoration of tubal integrity can preserve reproductive capability. Another conservative procedure involves partial salpingectomy with later anastomosis of proximal and distal segments of tube. Such attempts at conservation should be considered only in cases of unruptured ectopic pregnancy and only in consultation with surgeons experienced in and adept at such fertility procedures. The risk of recurrent ectopic pregnancy is definitely increased after any tubal surgery and such patients need special follow-up in subsequent pregnancies.

SUGGESTED READING
1. Breen JL: A 21 year survey of 654 ectopic pregnancies. Am J Obstet Gynecol 106:1004, 1970
2. Brenner PF: Ectopic pregnancy. JAMA 243:7, 673, 1980
3. Kitchin JD: Ectopic pregnancy: Current clinical trends. Am J Obstet Gynecol 134:870, 1979
4. Stromme WB: Conservative surgery for ectopic pregnancy, a 20 year review. Obstet Gynecol 41:215, 1973

F. Gary Cunningham, MD
David L. Hemsell, MD

Surgery for ruptured pelvic abscesses?

Correct dehydration, electrolytes, and acidosis when signs point to a leaking or ruptured pelvic abscess. Administer intensive high-dose broad-spectrum antimicrobials before attempting surgery, but operate immediately if the patient's initial condition is poor or begins to deteriorate.

Patients with ruptured tubo-ovarian or pelvic abscesses have a wide spectrum of signs and symptoms. The common denominator is that they always require immediate and aggressive therapy. A large volume of purulent material in the peritoneal cavity mandates prompt surgery; leakage may respond to intensive medical management alone or interval surgery.

Before the 1950s, when operative treatment was not the rule, 75% to 100% of patients with ruptured adnexal abscesses died. These devastating statistics prompted Collins and Mickal and their colleagues at Charity Hospital, New Orleans, and Vemeeren and TeLinde at Johns Hopkins Hospital to advocate drainage and adnexal extirpation.[1-3] This approach—coupled with new techniques for administering anesthesia, fluid replacement, and antimicrobials—has reversed the mortality/survival ratio (Table 9-1).

Who is at risk?

Patients with ruptured tubo-ovarian or pelvic abscesses make up only 0.2% to 0.3% of ad-

Table 9-1. History of surgical treatment for ruptured adnexal abscess

Author	Years	No.	Mortality(%)	Surgery*
Vemeeren and TeLinde[3]	1925–1944	22	90	1
(Johns Hopkins)	1945–1953	25	12	13
Pedowitz and Bloomfield[6]	<1947	16	100	1
(Brooklyn)	1947–1959	127	3.1	90
Mickal and Sellman[2]	1951–1959	54	11	94
(Charity Hospital, New Orleans)	1959–1966	55	3.7	

*Hysterectomy, bilateral salpingo-oophorectomy.

missions in teaching hospitals. Gynecologists in private practice probably encounter these problems even less frequently. Those with abscesses tend to be older and of lower parity than those with uncomplicated pelvic infections. A larger number are unfertile. Most ruptured abscesses occur in the third and fourth decades, but the reported age range is from preteens to the 70s.

Women who have had pelvic inflammatory disease are more likely to develop abscesses, but occasionally they complicate an initial episode of salpingitis. There is increasing evidence that IUD wearers are at higher risk. Those who have recently had hysterectomies may develop abscesses, usually following pelvic and cuff cellulitis. Table 9-2 gives the common physical findings associated with pelvic abscesses.

Signs and symptoms

A woman with a leaking or ruptured abscess appears ill and almost invariably complains of abdominal pain and, often, nausea, vomiting, and fever. Usually, she has had nonspecific lower abdominal or pelvic pain for several days, with a recent and sudden increase in intensity. Physical findings resemble peritonitis, the severity paralleling the severity of the illness. For example, overt rupture is accompanied by generalized peritonitis and dramatic clinical symptoms. But women in their mid-40s, and especially diabetics, may have little clinical evidence of peritonitis, despite unrelenting sepsis from large amounts of purulent material free in the peritoneal cavity. When only a small amount of material has leaked, symptoms and physical findings are generally less severe and are often confined to the pelvis or lower abdomen.

Sometimes a pelvic mass may be palpable, but frequently peritonitis precludes adequate examination. If the abscess is well confined, with leakage but little peritonitis, then it is more likely a mass will be felt. The patient may also be hypotensive, usually because the peritonitis depletes the intravascular volume. Suspect endotoxemia if the patient shows signs of hypothermia or significant pyrexia, as well as tachypnea and mental obtundation. Any of these findings should alert you that the patient is seriously ill.

Differential diagnosis

The following conditions in a young woman can mimic a leaking or ruptured abscess:

- Other adnexal pathology;
- A perforated appendix or one that is gangrenous, with either localized or generalized peritonitis;
- Purulent peritonitis with uncomplicated salpingitis;
- Inflammatory bowel conditions such as Crohn's disease;

Table 9-2. Common presenting symptoms with pelvic abscesses

	Ruptured	Leaking
Peritonitis	Generalized, appears toxic	Lower quadrants
Fever	Hyperthermia or hypothermia	Hyperthermia or normal
Volume status	Hypervolemia, hypotension	Usually isovolemic
Pelvic mass	Usually nonpalpable	Palpable
Ileus	Generalized	Segmental

- Complications of elective termination of pregnancy, usually following infection after perforation during suction curettage; and
- Uterine perforation during attempts to retrieve a lost IUD.

In the older woman, be suspicious when there is
- Bowel pathology;
- Appendicitis and any of its attendant complications;
- Perforation of a colonic diverticulum or of carcinoma;
- A gastric or duodenal ulcer; or
- Acute pancreatitis.

Aids in diagnosis and management

Ruptured pelvic abscesses are usually diagnosed clinically; however, some lab tests can help pinpoint associated conditions.

Hemogram. Leukocytosis with a shift to the left usually occurs with peritonitis; but leukopenia may suggest septicemia. The platelet count is usually normal, but thrombocytopenia may also accompany septicemia. The hematocrit will reflect dehydration and chronic infection, but if it is less than 30, there is probably concomitant blood loss. Request 6 to 8 units of cross-matched whole blood when you expect to operate.

Urinalysis. Acetonuria reflects dehydration and metabolic acidosis. Glucosuria should prompt you to check for diabetes, which may be precipitated by peritonitis or may actually mimic its signs and symptoms. Pyuria unaccompanied by bacilluria frequently indicates bacterial peritonitis. Although bacteriuria suggests urinary tract infection, this is almost never confused with intraperitoneal infection.

Serum chemistries and enzymes. At a minimum, determine serum sodium and potassium, to guide electrolyte replacement, and creatinine clearance, to assess renal function. With septicemia and peritonitis, invariably there is prerenal azotemia, and endotoxin is nephrotoxic. Hyperamylasemia suggests pancreatitis, usually a nonsurgical condition. Temporary abnormalities of liver function are frequent and suggest the presence of toxic hepatitis from septicemia.

Sonography. When you can't do an adequate pelvic examination, try sonography. Ultrasound can also help you measure palpated masses. Frequently, the sonolucent cavity will be smaller than the conglomerate tumor, because of edema and inflammation in the bowel wall and omentum adjacent to, or part of, a pelvic abscess.

X-rays. Plain and upright films of the abdomen usually are consistent with paralytic ileus. Free air may indicate a perforated, hollow viscus, but may also be from gas-forming organisms. Chest films are generally normal. A sympathetic pleural effusion may coexist with peritonitis, but when accompanied by an infiltrate, it suggests primary pulmonary damage from sepsis.

Culdocentesis. Culdocentesis will confirm hemoperitoneum, which can produce abdominal pain, fever, leukocytosis, and mild-to-moderate anemia. This procedure is a must in the older or diabetic woman whose history is consistent with any of these conditions, but whose examination results may not reflect the severity of the process. The procedure is not as helpful in the differential diagnosis when there is a palpable cul-de-sac abscess, or when there is generalized peritonitis.

Medical management

Immediate resuscitation is necessary to correct any systemic derangements resulting from severe infections. Replace fluids with balanced isotonic salt solution and continue until urine output is at least 30 ml/hour, and more optimally 60 ml/hour. It is not unusual for a woman to require 4 to 6 liters of saline or Ringer's solution to prompt such a diuresis. After the woman is isovolemic, determine the hematocrit again and, if it's less than 30, give whole blood or packed red blood cells. Before general anesthesia, add potassium as needed to correct hypokalemia. Rapid fluid replacement will correct metabolic acidosis.

Antimicrobial therapy. Begin broad-spectrum antimicrobial coverage and IV fluid replacement after taking blood and cul-de-sac samples for anaerobic and aerobic cultures. In our experience, any one of several regimens is suitable. Base your selection on your own experience and the patient's history of allergies (Table 9-3).

Adjunctive measures. The following procedures may also be necessary: central venous pressure determinations, nasogastric suction, supplemental oxygen, assisted ventilation for respiratory failure, or IV adrenal corticosteroids in pharmacologic doses. Methylprednisolone succinate, 15 to 30 mg/kg as an initial

Table 9-3. Antimicrobial regimens used for intra-abdominal sepsis

Drugs
1. Penicillin G—5 million units q 6 h
2. Cefamandole—2 gm q 4 h
3. Cefoxitin—2 gm q 4 h
4. Clindamycin—1,200 mg q 6 h
5. Chloramphenicol—50–100 mg/kg in four divided doses
6. Gentamicin—1.5 mg/kg q 8 h

Regimens
1 + 4 + 6
1 + 5 + 6
2 + 5
3 + 5

dose, repeated every 4 to 6 hours for four doses, should be considered if there is clinical evidence of septicemic shock.

Timing surgery

You may postpone surgery if there is a prompt response to medical management. For generalized peritonitis, however, plan celiotomy as soon as you have restored fluids and electrolytes and corrected metabolic acidosis.
Immediate laparotomy. When you must operate, make a lower midline incision with adequate preparation to allow for extension to the xiphoid. Upon entry, take peritoneal fluid for anaerobic and aerobic cultures. After identifying the site of the abscess, carefully dissect involved omentum and bowel to prevent perforation. Make sure all pelvic structures are completely free of contiguous structures before extirpating the adnexa or uterus. Because tissue planes are distorted and dissection is bloody, surgery will be safer and less blood will be lost if you isolate these structures before beginning a hysterectomy.

If both adnexa are involved, do a bilateral salpingo-oophorectomy. In many cases, hysterectomy is mandated because the uterus is involved with the abscess cavity. If there is substantial parametrial involvement, consider supracervical hysterectomy.

Bring multiple Penrose or Jackson-Pratt drains out through the vaginal cuff or through a posterior colpotomy incision if you don't remove the cervix or uterus. You may want to place indwelling abdominal catheters for postoperative irrigation, but we seldom use them. Before closing the abdomen, copiously irrigate the peritoneal cavity with warm saline, and remove all purulent material from the upper abdomen. Frequently, you may have to lyse adhesions and remove loculations of pus. Close the fascia with monofilament sutures using the Smead-Jones technique. Leave the skin and subcutaneous layers open and pack with fine-mesh gauze, soaked in povidone-iodine solution. Remove this three to four days later, and close the incision secondarily. Retention sutures may be beneficial.
Delayed operative intervention. In some cases, you can delay surgery safely for several days while you assess response to antimicrobial therapy. If peritonitis improves with three to five days of aggressive medical management, but no further, then operate. If fever and signs of peritonitis, albeit less severe, persist, then it is unlikely medical manage-

ment alone will succeed. Obviously, surgical exploration is indicated if the patient's condition worsens.

Interval surgery. Some leaks respond to aggressive medical and antimicrobial therapy, but usually you have to operate. We discharge patients who have been afebrile and asymptomatic for several days, place them on a regimen of oral antimicrobials, follow them closely, and schedule elective surgery in six to 12 weeks. If symptoms of infection occur before surgery is scheduled, we promptly readmit them, treat with IV antimicrobials, and perform surgery on the same admission—its urgency dictated by the patient's condition.

Most patients are best served by hysterectomy and bilateral adnexectomy. Conservative surgery is more appropriate for women who desire fertility. Ginsburg and colleagues at the Johns Hopkins Hospital found that after even conservative surgery for an unruptured abscess, fertility was poor.[4] Rivlin and Hunt, however, reported fertility *potential* in 42.5% and retained hormonal and menstrual function in 73.5% of 113 women after conservative surgery for generalized peritonitis due to ruptured abscesses.[5] Obviously, the extent of disease and the patient's overall medical condition and desire for future childbearing will influence the type of operation performed.

REFERENCES
1. Collins CG, Nix FG, Cerrha HT: Ruptured tuboovarian abscess. Am J Obstet Gynecol 72:820, 1956
2. Mickal A, Sellman AH: Management of tubo-ovarian abscess. Clin Obstet Gynecol 12:252, 1969
3. Vemeeren J, TeLinde RW: Intra-abdominal rupture of pelvic abscesses. Am J Obstet Gynecol 68:402, 1954
4. Ginsburg DS, Stern JL, Hamod KA, et al: Tubo-ovarian abscess: A retrospective review. Am J Obstet Gynecol 138:1055, 1980
5. Rivlin ME, Hunt JA: Ruptured tuboovarian abscess—Is hysterectomy necessary? Obstet Gynecol 50:518, 1977
6. Pedowitz P, Bloomfield RD: Ruptured adnexal abscess (tubo-ovarian) with generalized peritonitis. Am J Obstet Gynecol 88:721, 1964

Walter B. Jones, MD

How to cope with hemorrhage

10

Which patients are likely to hemorrhage? What techniques should you use to stop the bleeding and avoid recurrences? Is it possible to prevent bleeding?

The problem of vaginal hemorrhage is one that may confront the clinician at any time. Copious vaginal bleeding is a challenge not only to the oncologist but to the general gynecologist as well. In addition, the gynecologist is expected to manage the uterine hemorrhage that sometimes occurs with an underlying bleeding diathesis. The correct procedures, promptly applied, can usually stop the bleeding. Some hemorrhage can be prevented.

Patients likely to have problems
Hemorrhage can be defined as any bleeding that requires active treatment. It is often the first indication of a tumor in the vagina or cervix. It is seen most often in patients who have not consulted a physician since their last pregnancy, perhaps as long as 25 or 30 years ago. The vaginal bleeding is likely to be the first indication that a tumor exists.

Bleeding may also be the first sign of vaginal cancer in a young woman exposed in utero to diethylstilbestrol. But this has come to be the exception, because of the publicity given to the DES problem in recent years. Vaginal bleeding may be the first sign of sarcoma botryoides in very young children. Other patients at risk for severe vaginal hemorrhage are women with metastatic vaginal choriocarcinoma or metastases from primary ovarian, endometrial, and colonic tumors.

Hemorrhage from the uterus is often the hallmark of endometrial carcinoma, as every gynecologist knows only too well. It is also a characteristic sign of molar pregnancy. Occasionally, uterine hemorrhage may be a complication of acute leukemia, either as the initial sign of the disease or in patients who are undergoing chemotherapy. Such bleeding may also occur with aplastic anemia and von Willebrand disease.

Under certain circumstances, postoperative hemorrhage may be anticipated. Occasionally, a patient who has had cone biopsy of the cervix will have bleeding approximately 10 days to two weeks after the operation—the time when the catgut stitches dissolve. This type of bleeding is likely to result from faulty technique.

When hemorrhage complicates radical hysterectomy, it is usually because of incomplete hemostasis at the time of surgery. Patients who have undergone exenteration may also hemorrhage in the period immediately following operation. Most of these patients have cervix cancer unsuccessfully treated with radiation therapy. They also risk delayed hemorrhage months to years later. The source may simply be granulation tissue at the apex of the vaginal remnant, which begins to bleed spontaneously, or it may be the life-threatening rupture of hypogastric vessels.

Controlling the hemorrhage

Cervix and vaginal hemorrhage. You may choose among several methods to stop cervix and vaginal bleeding. The first step is, of course, to determine the cause. Modest bleeding from a vaginal tumor may be controlled by applying a silver nitrate stick to the area. Almost as simple, and perhaps more effective, is application of Monsel solution (ferric subsulfate), using a cotton swab or a soaked cotton ball, with direct pressure.

If the bleeding is copious, do suture ligation of the bleeding vessel with #0 chromic suture. If the vessel cannot be seen, suture the bleeding bed.

When this method is also unsuccessful, packing with a head-and-neck roll (gauze pack) saturated with acetone can be effective. When even this method fails, two alternatives are available—emergency irradiation or, as a last resort, ligation of the hypogastric vessels.

Ligating the hypogastrics interferes with the vascularization of the tumor-bearing area, and this may jeopardize future treatment of patients who will receive radiotherapy as definitive therapy. Use an external high-energy beam for bleeding tumors of the cervix or vagina. Give high dose fractions of 600 rads daily for three days through small 10 × 10-cm portals encompassing the tumor. Alternatively, intracavitary irradiation can be employed from either a radium or cesium source, at 1,500 to 2,000 mg/hour. Be ready to give blood transfusions as needed.

The correct treatment for a molar pregnancy is to evacuate the uterus with suction during an infusion of an oxytoxic agent. Then give a uterotropic agent such as ergotrate. At one time, hysterotomy was the procedure of choice when the uterus was enlarged, but today evacuation can be accomplished safely from below, regardless of the size of the uterus. In metastatic trophoblastic disease, we sometimes see a mass in the vagina. Such lesions should never be biopsied or excised, because of the bleeding danger.

One patient with a vaginal metastasis, correctly treated with chemotherapy, responded with disappearance of the mass and a drop in hCG titer, though not to normal values. She failed to return for recommended follow-up and, six months later, staff at another hospital informed us that the woman had been admitted and was hemorrhaging. She was transferred to our hospital, still bleeding profusely from a recurrence of the vaginal metastasis. We started transfusions in both arms, and attempted to stanch the flow with cautery and packing. Both methods were unsuccessful, as was suturing. The tumor had a soft, spongy consistency; it was like trying to suture a pudding. We ligated the hypogastric arteries and, immediately after the operation, irradiated the vaginal tumor.

We then treated this patient with the combination chemotherapy that had been successful the first time. Within two months her titer returned to normal and the vaginal tumor completely disappeared. Unfortunately, the patient again failed to return for follow-up appointments.

Endometrial hemorrhage. Diagnostic D & C can also be therapeutic for an endometrial hemorrhage. If the D & C fails to stop the bleeding, the uterus can be packed. Begin by packing both cornua, then pack the central cavity. Packing should be left in place for

48 hours, then removed slowly and carefully. When this technique fails, try external radiation therapy. Should the hemorrhage continue, add intracavitary irradiation with radium or cesium.

One patient with severe uterine hemorrhage caused by aplastic anemia responded atypically. When the original packing was removed, she again began to hemorrhage; the uterus had to be repacked. Then, two weeks later, she started to bleed again. Remember that this patient's basic problem was a hemorrhagic diathesis, not a gynecologic condition. She was also bleeding from other orifices— bladder, rectum, mouth. Once again, the uterus was packed and a transfusion with platelets and other coagulation factors given. About a week later, the patient became febrile. Because we thought infection might be developing, we removed the packing. A pack left in place too long in a granulocytopenic patient makes infection always a possibility.

Postexenteration hemorrhage. Hemorrhage after exenteration may be the result of previous intensive radiation therapy that produced tissue necrosis, or recurrent tumor. It is sometimes possible to visualize the source of the bleeding, when a perineal opening remains. Occasionally, the bleeding can be controlled from below by applying a clamp or a hemoclip to the vessel. The clamp can be left in place for 24 to 48 hours, if hemostasis cannot be achieved otherwise, or until adequate replacement transfusion has been carried out, if exploratory surgery is planned. However, clamping the vessel from below may be unsuccessful, particularly in older women whose vessels may have become fragile as the result of arteriosclerosis. The only certain method of controlling such bleeding is to perform a laparotomy and stop the bleeding from within.

Bleeding from the distal stump of the hypogastric artery or pelvic floor vein may be severe. You can usually identify the source of the bleeding by suctioning to remove fresh blood and following the suction catheter down to the source of the bleeding. If you have found the source, put a large hemoclip on it. If not, ligate the vascular bed with silk sutures. As a last resort, apply a pelvic pack, using a head-and-neck roll.

While there is no way to prevent bleeding after exenteration, there are warning signs. A history of even minimal bleeding from the perineum may portend severe bleeding episodes. Watch for evidence of any bleeding at all. Seek the source immediately; don't wait for active bleeding.

Hemorrhage in acute leukemia. For patients with acute leukemia following chemotherapy, or for those who have other hemorrhagic diatheses, D & C is not recommended. Vaginal bleeding can often be controlled by means of therapeutic amenorrhea. First, give medroxyprogesterone acetate, 10 mg every 4 hours, for rapid cessation of bleeding. Once active bleeding diminishes, give a combination pill containing a potent progestin such as Ovral. In leukemic patients, continue this therapy until the bone marrow recovers sufficiently from the effects of the cytotoxic drugs that the threat of blood loss from normal menstrual flow no longer need be feared. There is no objection to continuing therapeutic amenorrhea throughout the treatment period.

Preventing hemorrhage

Many bleeding episodes occur because patients did not consult a physician in time. Early treatment of cervix and vaginal cancers usually makes such episodes unlikely.

Avoid biopsy of a metastatic focus of choriocarcinoma in the vagina. This can cause uncontrollable, often fatal, hemorrhage.

Figure 10-1. Relationship between hemorrhage and platelet count*

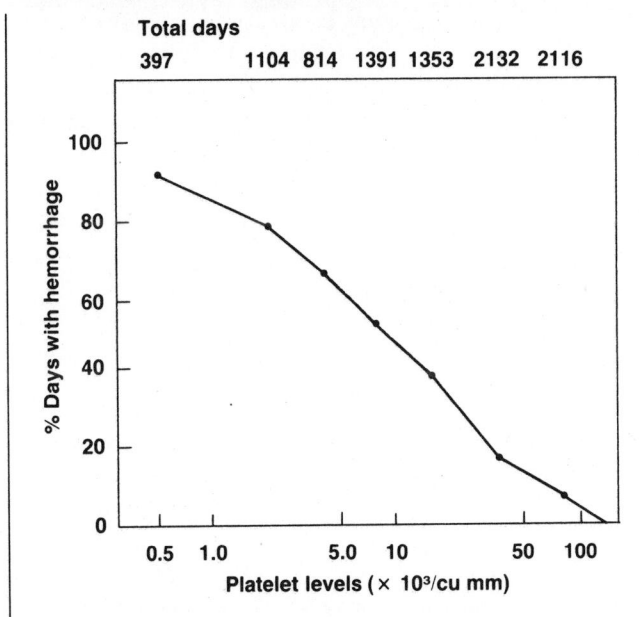

Total days: 397   1104   814   1391   1353   2132   2116

[Graph: % Days with hemorrhage vs Platelet levels (× 10^3/cu mm)]

Curve shows percentage of days with hemorrhage in a 92-patient group, correlated with platelet readings. Low—and falling—counts indicate need for intervention.

*Modified from Gaydos LA, Freireich EJ, Mantel N.[2]

In solid tumors,[1] as well as acute leukemia,[2] low platelet levels may predict bleeding episodes (see Figure 10-1). If the platelet count is in the low-normal range and falling fast, give platelets immediately and be prepared to intervene surgically, if necessary.

REFERENCES
1. Belt RJ, Leite C, Haas CD, et al: Incidence of hemorrhage complications in patients with cancer. JAMA 239:2571, 1978
2. Gaydos LA, Freireich EJ, Mantel N: The quantitative relationship between platelet count and hemorrhage in patients with acute leukemia. N Engl J Med 266:905, 1962

Leon Speroff, MD

Managing anovulatory bleeding medically

11

Selecting the correct therapy involves choosing between intense progestin-estrogen combination medication and high doses of estrogen. Appropriate biopsy may be indicated.

Categorizing endometrial bleeding by descriptive terms, such as hypomenorrhea, hypermenorrhea, polymenorrhea, menorrhagia, and metrorrhagia, only serves to complicate clinical management. These are terms designed to tax one's memory. It is more straightforward and helpful to have a general understanding of normal and abnormal bleeding.

The most reproducible indication of menstrual function, in terms of quantity and duration, is the postovulatory estrogen-progesterone withdrawal-bleeding response. This response is so dependable that many women, over the years, come to expect a certain characteristic flow pattern. Any slight deviation may be a cause for concern on the patient's part and may require strong reassurance from the physician. Significant deviation requires evaluation for a local or systemic problem. A thorough history and physical examination are usually sufficient for evaluating teenagers. However, adult patients often require appropriate biopsies, including one of the current vacuum techniques for endometrial sampling.

Defining the problem

Dysfunctional uterine bleeding can be defined as the bleeding manifestations of anovulatory cycles. This type of bleeding can result from systemic problems, such as hypothyroidism, obesity, and liver disease, or from psychogenic problems, such as mild anorexia nervosa. Regardless of the cause, anovulatory cycles may produce abnormal bleeding patterns and often can be managed without surgical intervention. Indeed, failure to control vaginal bleeding with medical therapy strongly suggests a pathologic condition within the reproductive tract.

Abnormal patterns include:
- Excessive or prolonged cyclic bleeding;
- Delayed menses followed by heavy or prolonged flow;
- Premenstrual and postmenstrual spotting;
- Intermenstrual bleeding.

There are two common major categories of dysfunctional endometrial bleeding. The first, *estrogen breakthrough bleeding*, is characteristic of anovulation. The amount of circulating estrogen and fluctuations in the blood level determine the type of bleeding. Relatively low amounts of estrogen yield intermittent spotting, which may be prolonged, but the flow is generally light. High levels of estrogen and sustained availability lead to prolonged periods of amenorrhea, followed by acute and often profuse bleeds with excessive loss of blood. High levels of estrogen are most often associated with polycystic ovary syndrome, immaturity of the hypothalamic-pituitary-ovarian axis in teenagers, and late anovulation in perimenopausal women. Without growth-limiting progesterone and periods of desquamation, the endometrium attains an abnormal height but no competent structural support. This tissue is fragile and suffers spontaneous breakage and bleeding.

The second type, *progestational breakthrough bleeding*, is encountered in patients who are anovulatory as the result of taking progestin medication, such as birth control pills, progestin therapy for endometriosis, or treatment with depot forms of progestin. Without sufficient estrogen, continuous progestational impact on the endometrium yields intermittent bleeding of variable duration, which can be heavy at times.

Estrogen and progestational breakthrough bleeding lack self-limitation, the single most important property of the estrogen-progesterone withdrawal bleed that follows the ovulatory cycle. There are three reasons for the self-limiting character of ovulatory bleeding:

- It is a universal endometrial event. The onset and conclusion of menses are related to a precise sequence of hormonal events, and menstrual changes begin almost simultaneously in all segments of the endometrium.
- The endometrial tissue that has responded to a sequence of estrogen and progesterone is structurally stable and the events leading to ischemic disintegration of the endometrium are orderly and progressive.
- The vasomotor response involved in stopping menstrual flow is a consequence of the events that start menstrual bleeding following estrogen-progesterone stimulation. Waves of vasoconstriction initiate the ischemic event to provoke menses; prolonged vasoconstriction, abetted by the stasis associated with endometrial collapse, enables clotting factors to seal off exposed bleeding sites. In the subsequent cycle, the resumed stimulation of rising estrogen levels adds to the healing effect.

Choosing the therapy

After evaluation and examination, including biopsies if appropriate, the immediate objective of medical therapy for anovulatory bleeding is to restore the natural controlling influences—universal, synchronous endometrial events, structural stability, and vasomotor rhythmicity. Therapy involves an initial choice between high-dose progestin-estrogen combination medication and high doses of estrogen.

Any brand of progestin-estrogen oral contraceptives can control bleeding rapidly and easily. Administer one pill q.i.d. for five to seven days. Continue this therapy even though flow usually ceases within 12 to 24 hours. If flow does not clearly diminish, re-evaluate other diagnostic possibilities, such as polyps, incomplete abortion, and neoplasia, by examination under anesthesia and D & C. If flow does diminish rapidly, the remainder of the week of treatment can be devoted to evaluating causes of anovulation, hemorrhagic tendencies, and iron or blood replacement.

The four-pills-a-day therapy induces structural rigidity intrinsic to the compact pseudodecidual reaction. Continued random breakdown of formerly fragile tissue is avoided and blood loss is stopped. However, a relatively large amount of tissue remains to react to withdrawal of the medication. Consequently, the patient must be warned to anticipate a heavy, perhaps severely cramping, flow two to four days after stopping therapy.

Continued control of bleeding requires maintaining cyclic combination birth control medication. Each successive cycle serves to prevent any regrowth that might be caused by unopposed estrogen and allows orderly regression of excessive endometrial height to normal controllable levels.

For the patient who does not require contraception and whose endometrial tissue has been reduced to normal height, discontinue the pill and start monthly progestin therapy. Recent studies in England found that postmenopausal women needed 10 days of progestational therapy to prevent hyperplasia and endometrial adenocarcinoma.[1] Therefore, it seems wise to apply this duration of therapy to the younger anovulatory woman. Accordingly, medroxyprogesterone acetate, 10 mg orally, is given the first 10 days of every month. This induces a reasonable flow two to seven days after the last pill and prevents excessive endometrial buildup. Regular shedding and the need to form new tissue each month prevent prolonged stimulation and development of hyperplasia. If bleeding occurs at an unexpected time, spontaneous ovulation must be suspected.

Spontaneous ovulation in the anovulatory patient is possible and unpredictable. Since there is no evidence that birth control pills increase risk of secondary amenorrhea, the need for contraception takes precedence. In a patient who requires contraception, it is prudent to maintain pill medication.

Bleeding manifestations are frequently associated with low estrogen stimulation. There is usually intermittent vaginal spotting, and endometrial biopsy yields little tissue. Progestin treatment has no beneficial effect, because a tissue base is lacking on which the progestin may exert its organizational and strengthening action. This is also true of anovulatory patients in whom prolonged hemorrhage leaves little residual tissue. Give such patients high-dose estrogen therapy—conjugated estrogens, 25 mg IV every 4 hours, until bleeding diminishes. Usually, treatment is maintained for 24 hours. If this high-dose estrogen therapy does not significantly diminish flow within 12 to 24 hours, D & C is necessary. If blood flow does diminish, initiate therapy with combination oral contraceptives. When bleeding is not excessive and IV therapy is not practical, a program of oral high-dose estrogen medication may be used: 10 mg conjugated estrogens for seven days, followed by combination birth control pills.

Two problems clinicians frequently encounter are associated with progestin breakthrough bleeding: the bleeding encountered with birth control pills and that related to treatment regimens using oral or depot forms of progestin. When there is insufficient endogenous and exogenous estrogen, the endometrium becomes shallow. It is composed almost exclusively of pseudodecidual stroma and blood vessels with minimal glands. This type of endometrium is also fragile and may break down. Breakthrough bleeding in the first few months of treatment is best managed by encouragement and reassurance. If necessary, even this early pattern can be treated with exogenous estrogen.

It is helpful to explain to the patient that this bleeding represents tissue breakdown as the endometrium readjusts from its usual thick state to the relatively thin state promoted by the progestin therapy. If bleeding occurs just before the end of a pill cycle, it can be managed by having the patient stop the pills, wait seven days, and start a new cycle. If breakthrough bleeding is prolonged or distressing, it can be controlled by a short course of exogenous estrogen. Give conjugated estrogens, 2.5 mg, or ethinylestradiol, 20 µg, daily for seven days, no matter where the patient is in her pill or treatment cycle. Have her adhere to the pill-taking schedule. Usually one course of estrogen solves the problem. Recurrence of breakthrough bleeding is unusual, but if it does recur, another seven-day course of estrogen is effective.

Table 11-1. Principal points of medical therapy for anovulatory bleeding

- Evaluate by history and physical examination.
- Begin intense progestin-estrogen therapy and maintain it for seven days.
- Continue cyclic low-dose oral contraceptives for at least three months.
- For premenopausal, sexually active women, continue oral contraception.
- If contraception is unnecessary, induce progestational withdrawal bleeding on a monthly basis with medroxyprogesterone acetate, 10 mg for the first 10 days of each month.
- Give high-dose estrogen therapy—25 mg conjugated estrogen IV every 4 hours—under the following conditions:
    if bleeding has been prolonged;
    if the biopsy yields minimal tissue;
    if the patient is on progestin medication.
- If this medical therapy produces no response in 12 to 24 hours, proceed with D & C.

Increasing the dose of the progestational agent does not correct irregular bleeding. The progestin component of the pill will always dominate; doubling the number of pills doubles the progestational impact, with its decidualizing, atrophic effect on the endometrium. Adding extra estrogen while keeping the progestin dose unchanged is logical and effective.

If a patient has recurrent bleeding despite repeated medical therapy, you must suspect submucous myomas or endometrial polyps. Even thorough curettage can miss such pathology and further diagnostic study may be helpful. Either hysterosalpingography, with slow instillations of dye and careful fluoroscopic examination, or hysteroscopy may reveal a myoma or polyp. These conditions are particularly likely in the puzzling case of a patient with abnormal bleeding and ovulatory cycles.

REFERENCE
1. Paterson MEL, Wade-Evans T, Sturdee OW, et al: Endometrial disease after treatment with oestrogens and progestogens in the climacteric. Br Med J 1:822, 1980

Edward J. Quilligan, MD

Fetal bradycardia: Watch or deliver?

When scalp blood values are available, deliver the baby as soon as possible if the pH is less than 7.20 or if the trend is toward increasing acidosis. Without a scalp pH, it's better to overdiagnose and deliver the baby when the FHR pattern shows severe variable or late decelerations.

There is ample evidence that bradycardia is frequently associated with decreased oxygenation of the fetus.[1,2] But which episodes of bradycardia are associated with how much hypoxia and what is the best way to manage suspected hypoxia? In general, the following conditions indicate increased fetal hypoxia: baseline tachycardia, when the mother has no fever; decreased FHR variability, when the mother hasn't been given drugs; and meconium staining of the amniotic fluid.

Basic guidelines

Benson and others find a high false-negative rate for the traditional indicator of fetal distress—any ausculted heart rate decrease below 100 beats per minute (bpm), lasting beyond a uterine contraction.[3] Hon places the diagnosis of fetal distress on a firmer footing when he describes the periodic changes in FHR associated with uterine contractions.[4] He classifies decelerations as early, late, and variable—according to their onset in relation

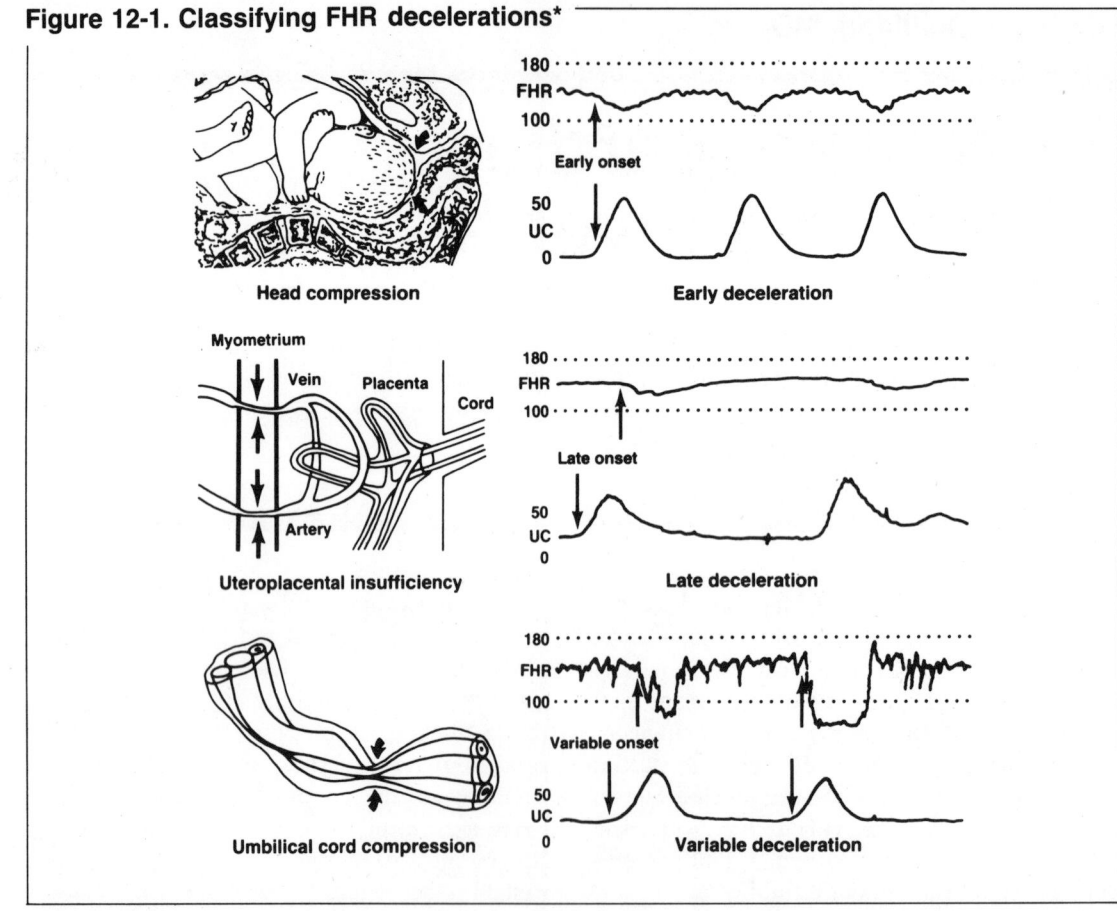

Figure 12-1. Classifying FHR decelerations*

Head compression — Early deceleration

Uteroplacental insufficiency — Late deceleration

Umbilical cord compression — Variable deceleration

*Adapted from Hon HE.[4]

to the onset of the uterine contraction—and characterizes their waveforms. The early and late are reverse images of the contraction waveform, with a slow decrease and recovery, and the variable deceleration has a rapid descent and recovery. When this analysis is used, head compression seems associated with early deceleration, uteroplacental insufficiency with late deceleration, and umbilical cord compression with variable deceleration (Figure 12-1).

Caldeyro-Barcia's group in Montevideo combines early and early variable decelerations into the type I dip and late plus late variable decelerations into the type II dip.[5] Late decelerations, severe variable decelerations, and type II dips are potentially ominous because these patterns have been associated with a decrease in fetal arterial oxygen tension. The clinical significance of these patterns is modified by the baseline FHR, the variability of FHR, and meconium staining.

Managing specific cases of bradycardia

The studies of Haverkamp and co-workers raise doubts about the value of continuous fetal heart rate monitoring for predicting the baby's condition.[6,7] But we find the technique valuable, especially when backed up with blood sampling.

When fetal scalp blood sampling facilities are available, follow the monitoring protocol shown in Figure 12-2. When ominous patterns are present, give the mother 100% oxygen by mask and change her position to right or left lateral (or dorsal), depending on the position she was in when the deceleration was picked up. Correct any factors that may be responsible for reduced uterine blood flow. If the mother is receiving oxytocin and the uterine contractions are too frequent, stop the drug. If she becomes hypotensive following conduction anesthesia, give 500 to 1,000 ml lactated Ringer's solution, put her in a lateral position, and give 25 mg ephedrine if the blood pressure remains low.

If a normal pattern results, carefully observe the patient for further changes, but obtain a fetal scalp sample if the deceleration pattern persists despite corrective measures. If the pattern is one of severe late deceleration (FHR < 80 bpm) without variability, proceed to immediate delivery.

If the scalp sample indicates pH is greater than 7.25, continue to observe unless the FHR pattern worsens, for example, if mild

Figure 12-2. Using FHR and scalp blood pH to assess fetal bradycardia

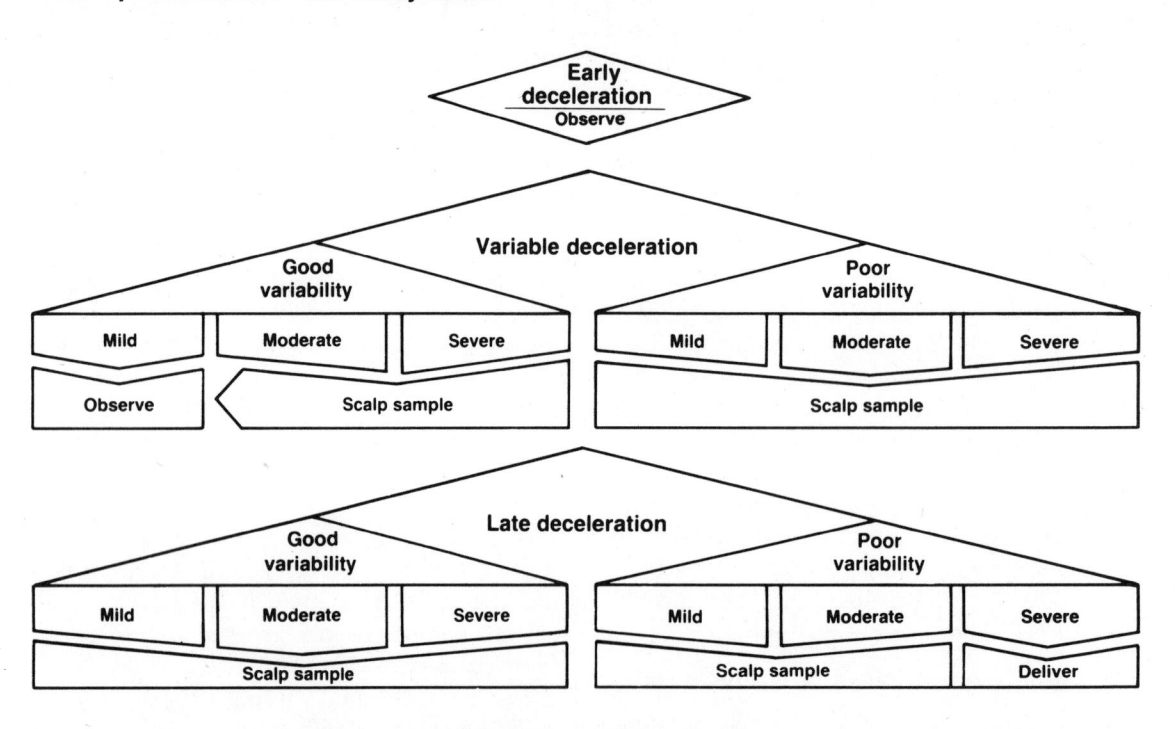

```
                    Early
                 deceleration
                   Observe

                Variable deceleration
         Good                        Poor
       variability                 variability
   Mild  Moderate  Severe    Mild  Moderate  Severe
  Observe   Scalp sample         Scalp sample

                  Late deceleration
         Good                        Poor
       variability                 variability
   Mild  Moderate  Severe    Mild  Moderate  Severe
        Scalp sample          Scalp sample   Deliver
```

Scalp sample: >7.25, repeat in 30 minutes; 7.20-7.25, repeat in 15 minutes; <7.20, deliver; trend toward increasing acidosis with repeat samples, deliver.

Figure 12-3. Using FHR to assess fetal bradycardia

```
                    ┌─────────────┐
                    │    Early    │
                    │ deceleration│
                    │   Observe   │
                    └─────────────┘

              Variable deceleration
        Examine vagina for umbilical cord prolapse

         Good variability                    Poor variability

    Mild      Moderate      Severe      Mild    Moderate    Severe

  Observe   Observe with  Observe with Observe  Observe with position
            position      position              change for 15 minutes
            change and    change and
            O₂ for 60     maternal O₂
            minutes       for 30 minutes


                        Late deceleration

         Good variability              Thick meconium
                                       or poor variability

    Mild      Moderate      Severe      Mild    Moderate    Severe

  Observe with maternal   Observe with  Observe  Observe    Deliver
  O₂ for 60 minutes       maternal O₂   with     with       immediately
                          for 30        maternal maternal
                          minutes       O₂ for   O₂ for
                                        15       10–15
                                        minutes  minutes
```

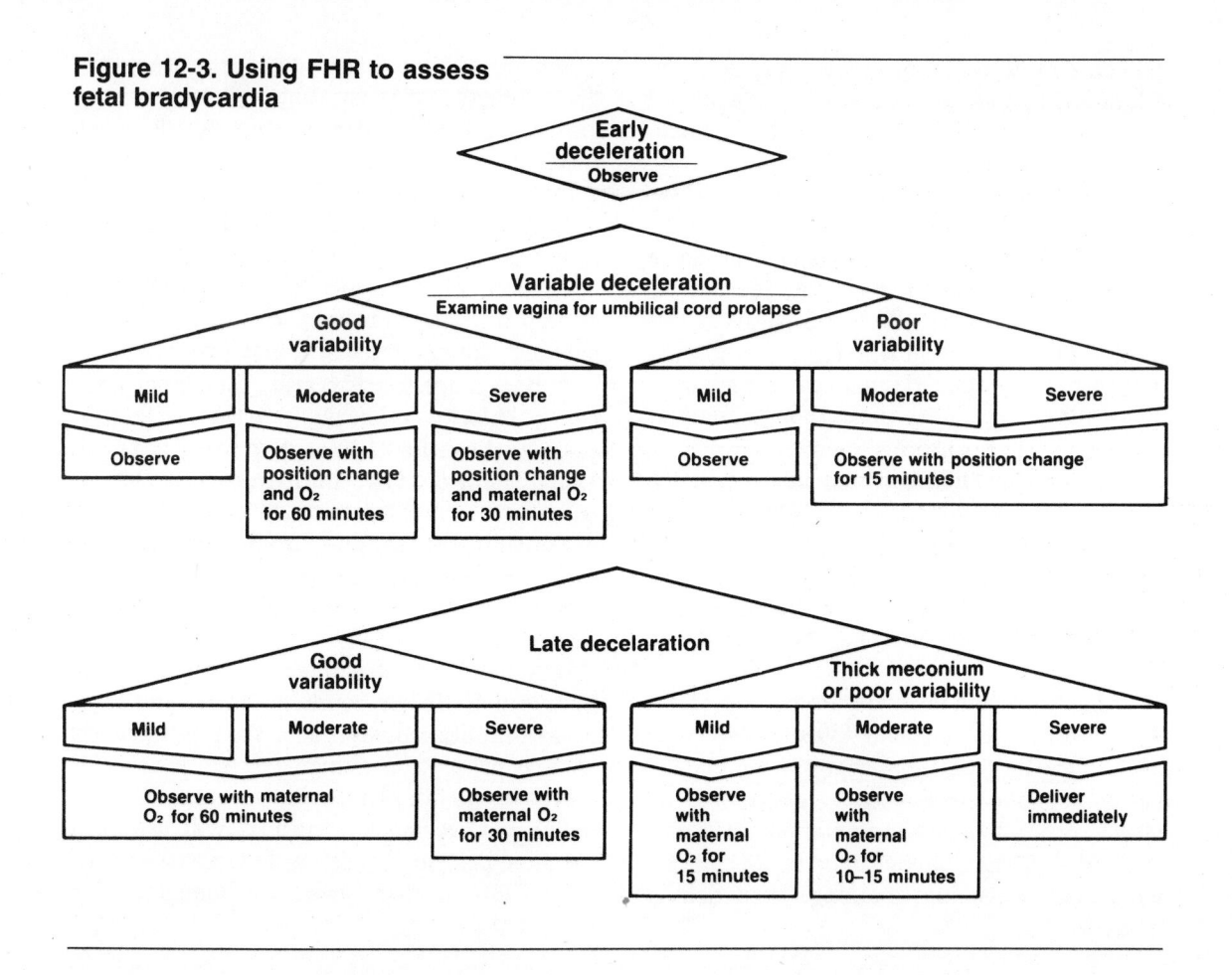

late decelerations become moderate late decelerations. Take another sample 30 minutes later, unless the FHR has returned to normal. If a more ominous pattern develops, obtain scalp blood immediately and deliver the infant if the pH has decreased.

If the pH is 7.20 to 7.25, take another scalp sample in 15 minutes and deliver the baby if the pH is going down. If the initial pH is less than 7.20, deliver immediately. Scalp sampling is useful if the FHR pattern is unclear or if there is no variability, even though ominous decelerations are absent.

When scalp sampling is unavailable (Figure 12-3), err on the side of overdiagnosing fetal distress. With good FHR variability, observe and try to correct ominous patterns for 30 minutes. If there is no amelioration of severe variable or late decelerations, then deliver the baby.

If there are mild or moderate late decelerations, observe for an hour (30 minutes, with severe late decelerations) when there is good variability, no baseline tachycardia, and no meconium staining of the amniotic fluid. But if the FHR is flat, particularly in association with thick meconium staining, then deliver immediately.

Sometimes, the fetus develops a bradycardia that lasts more than 2 minutes and that begins like a variable deceleration but does not return to baseline. In such cases, move to the delivery/section room and be prepared for an emergency delivery unless the FHR returns to normal within 5 minutes. Three or more decelerations of this type call for delivery. Although the baby is usually well at the time of delivery, there have been some deaths.

For prolonged bradycardia following paracervical block anesthesia, give the mother oxygen to breathe (100% at 5 liters/minute). Don't begin delivery until the FHR has returned to normal for 15 to 20 minutes.

Continuous baseline bradycardia (< 100 bpm) occasionally occurs with fetal heart block. You can distinguish this pattern from a maternal heart rate that is being picked up through a dead fetus if you record fetal and maternal ECGs or count maternal and fetal rates simultaneously. If a true fetal heart block is present, as demonstrated by lack of P waves in the fetal ECG, don't treat until after delivery. Occasionally, the fetus will develop a terminal baseline bradycardia associated with a flat FHR. In such a case, you should deliver immediately.

REFERENCES
1. Myers RE, Mueller-Heubach E, Adamsons K: Predictability of the state of fetal oxygenation from a quantitative analysis of the components of late deceleration. Am J Obstet Gynecol 115:1083, 1973
2. Kubli FW, Hon EH, Khazin AF, et al: Observations on fetal heart rate and pH in the human fetus during labor. Am J Obstet Gynecol 104:1190, 1969
3. Benson RC, Shubeck F, Deutschberger J, et al: Fetal heart rate as a predictor of fetal distress. A report from the collaborative project. Obstet Gynecol 32:259, 1968
4. Hon HE: Observations on pathologic fetal bradycardia. Am J Obstet Gynecol 77:1084, 1959
5. Schwarcz RL, Belizan JM, Cifuerites JR, et al: Fetal and maternal monitoring in spontaneous labors and in elective inductions. Am J Obstet Gynecol 120:356, 1974
6. Haverkamp AD, Thompson HE, McFee JG, et al: The evaluation of continuous fetal heart rate monitoring in high risk pregnancy. Am J Obstet Gynecol 125:310, 1976
7. Haverkamp AD, Orleans M, Langendoerfer S, et al: A controlled trial of the differential effects of intrapartum monitoring. Am J Obstet Gynecol 134:399, 1979

Frederick P. Zuspan, MD
Kathryn J. Zuspan, MD

Strategies for controlling eclampsia

Once your diagnosis is definite, begin magnesium sulfate therapy. It offers 99% maternal survival and greater than 90% fetal salvage. The authors outline their regimen.

The word means to strike forth or suddenly appear, but eclampsia rarely develops suddenly. Only our inability to perceive its subtle progression impedes early diagnosis. A catabolic disease that develops gradually, eclampsia is part of a continuum characterized by the increasing edema, acute hypertension, and proteinuria of preeclampsia, followed finally by the generalized eclamptic convulsion (Table 13-1). Because the severity varies with a bell-shaped curve, some eclamptic patients are actually less ill than some who have severe preeclampsia.

Incidence figures are difficult to determine accurately. It probably ranges from 1.2 to 2.6 per 1,000 deliveries. Maternal mortality, worldwide, is between 0 and 17%; fetal mortality, between 10% and 37%. Among obstetric problems with potential for loss of life, it is thus one of the most hazardous. Management goals must be directed at controlling the hypertension and alleviating symptoms, since the underlying cause is unknown.

Once eclampsia develops, it is a medical emergency that must be given the highest priority by a skilled health-care team. Before

Table 13-1. Pathophysiology of eclampsia

Normal pregnancy	Mild preeclampsia	Severe preeclampsia	Eclampsia
▲ Aldosterone ▲ Sodium retention ▲ Fluid retention ▲ Weight gain	▲ Cardiovascular reactivity ▲ Vasospasm ▲ Blood pressure Uteroplacental bed Vascular occlusion	Fibrin deposition Renal lesion Proteinuria ▼ Vascular volume CNS irritability ▲ Amines ▼ PG dilators	Convulsion

that, the aim of therapy is to prevent preeclampsia from progressing to the characteristic convulsions. The ultimate aim, of course, is prevention of maternal complications and delivery of a healthy baby.

Pathophysiology of acute hypertension of pregnancy

Vasospasms at the arteriole level produce hypertension and, ultimately, decrease uterine blood flow. Normally, the pregnant patient is resistant to pressor agents. But in preeclampsia, the patient develops increased vascular sensitivity.

Patients with moderate to severe preeclampsia cannot handle ingested sodium appropriately, because of altered renal function. As preeclampsia develops, a renal vascular lesion, glomeruloendotheliosis, appears. Glomerular function diminishes and glomerular filtration rate declines from the normal 100 ml/minute or higher. This renal lesion disappears after delivery. It is usually associated with a significant proteinuria—more than 2+.

There is decreased volume in the vascular compartment because more solutes are present in the third space. Keep this decreased blood volume in mind as you follow the patient through serial hematocrit determinations. These will be higher than normal.

CNS alterations proceed from hyperactive reflexes, to clonus, to a generalized seizure. Fetal and maternal mortality correlate with the number of seizures.

Diagnosis and complications

The only difference between eclampsia and severe preeclampsia is seizure and the fact that the eclamptic patient is usually sicker. The common clinical signs of both are weight gain of more than 5 to 6 lb in a week, often accompanied by headaches, epigastric pain, and disturbed vision, especially scotomata. Test results that are diagnostic include:

- Systolic blood pressure of 160 or diastolic pressure of 110, recorded twice at 6-hour intervals with the patient at bedrest;
- Proteinuria reading of 5 gm in 24 hours or 3+ to 4+ on dipstick;
- Oliguria—urinary output of less than 400 ml in 24 hours;
- Cerebral or eye disturbances, including eyeground changes; and
- Pulmonary edema or cyanosis.

A generalized seizure, associated with edema, hypertension, and (usually) proteinuria, confirms the diagnosis.

The three most serious complications are cerebrovascular accident or cerebral edema, placental abruption with or without hypofibrinogenemia or disseminated intravascular coagulation, and fetal death. Death is a risk for the mother when the brain, the liver and hemopoietic system, or the kidneys are compromised. Complications in the brain include cerebral hemorrhage; in the liver, disseminated intravascular coagulation and periportal necrosis; in the kidneys, glomeruloendotheliosis and severe oliguria.

Choosing the treatment

Therapy is much the same, whether the patient has eclampsia or severe preeclampsia. The extent of therapy is dictated by the degree of illness, and how worried the healthcare team is.

Regimens vary from country to country and from specialty to specialty. In the U.K., clinicians use epidural anesthesia to control blood pressure; they treat convulsions with diazepam and edema with IV diuretics. In the U.S., clinicians control blood pressure with

101

IV hydralazine and treat convulsions with therapeutic doses of magnesium sulfate.[1,2] No one really knows whether the disease is the same in Europe and the U.S. We believe prominent academicians influence the mode of practice in their countries.

Here in the U.S., over the past 25 years, Pritchard and Zuspan have been major proponents of parenteral magnesium sulfate. Pritchard administers $MgSO_4$ IM while Zuspan prefers the IV route. Their methods and results are basically identical. Both have achieved 90% fetal salvage and reduced maternal mortality to near zero levels. These results, reported in 1965 (Zuspan and Ward) and 1967 (Pritchard and Stone), were the best in the world literature and remain so.[3,4]

The case for magnesium therapy

Magnesium is the fourth most common cation (positively charged ion) in the body and the second most plentiful intracellular cation. Administered parenterally, it is excreted almost entirely in the urine; only 1% to 2% is recovered in the feces. Magnesium activates a host of enzyme systems critical to cellular metabolism and is a required cofactor for oxidative metabolism in vitro. Magnesium and calcium have a complex interdependent influence on the excitability of the neuromuscular junction.

In pharmacologic doses, magnesium may have a curariform action on the neuromuscular junction, interfering with the release of acetylcholine from motor-nerve terminals. Another hypothesis is that replacing calcium with magnesium changes membrane potential. This change would prevent convulsions by altering neuromuscular transmission and the excitability of the motor-nerve terminal.

Many investigators believe that magnesium excess at concentrations between 8 and 10 mEq/liter is expressed clinically by hypoactive deep tendon reflexes. Respiratory paralysis occurs at concentrations greater than 13 to 15 mEq/liter. Concentrations in excess of 25 mEq/liter produce cardiac arrest.

The term "magnesium sulfate" refers to the hydrated form, $MgSO_4 \cdot 7H_2O$. The anhydrous salt contains twice as much magnesium as the hydrated. Magnesium sulfate has been used since 1906 for the treatment of both preeclampsia and eclampsia. Lazard first popularized IV magnesium sulfate in 1925. Eastman is credited with establishing the current IM regimen (Table 13-2). The regimens listed in the table are only guidelines.

Table 13-2. Specific eclampsia therapy

Magnesium sulfate

Loading dose, 4 gm, over 10 minutes
Then 1 to 2 gm per hour by infusion device

Antihypertensive drugs
(if diastolic blood pressure is over 100)

Hydralazine, 5 mg bolus, IV
Then by regulated delivery system, IV

Constant MD and nurse supervision

Early decision for delivery

In planning therapy, take into consideration the patient's body weight and urinary excretions, as well as the clinical severity of the disease. Use reflexes, respiration, and urinary output as bioassay parameters to monitor the patient. Reflexes should be hypoactive but present, respiration at least 14 per minute, and urine output more than 100 ml every 4 hours.

Sibai and colleagues found convulsions recurred in 1% of eclamptic patients treated with Zuspan's regimen—a loading dose of 4 gm IV followed by a maintenance dose consisting of 1 gm/hour IV.[1]

Prevalent misconceptions are that $MgSO_4$ in very minimal amounts crosses the blood-brain barrier, and that it has hypotensive qualities. Magnesium sulfate does cross the placenta and is present in essentially the same concentrations in cord blood as in maternal blood. It is excreted by the fetus within 48 hours with no ill effect. It is not a hypotensive agent, though it does decrease intrinsic resistance in uterine vessels and may occasionally cause a transient decline in blood pressure, which soon returns to baseline levels. Whether magnesium also decreases uterine activity is being debated. It may do so in some individuals, causing a problem in induction of labor.

Recommended treatment

Once eclampsia develops, both mother and fetus require intensive care. The following regimen should result in less than 1% maternal mortality and greater than 90% fetal salvage.

During convulsion—
■ Place padded tongue blade in mouth.
■ Give magnesium sulfate 4 to 6 gm IV over 4 to 10 minutes to control the convulsions. Do *not* use diazepam or sodium amobarbital, because they depress mother and fetus.

After convulsion—

■ Insert a plastic airway and give the patient oxygen.
■ Place patient in Trendelenburg position.
■ Suction passages to remove secretions.
■ If the stomach is full, empty stomach with nasogastric tube and instill antacid before removing the tube.
■ Start IV with 5% dextrose in 0.25 N saline to replace urine output and insensible loss. Use 5% dextrose in 0.5 N saline if electrolyte levels are abnormal.
■ Insert Foley catheter and record intake and output every hour.
■ Order 24-hour urinalysis for protein, creatinine, and estriol.
■ Check urine for specific gravity and for protein every 6 to 8 hours.
■ Check serial hematocrits every 6 to 8 hours.
■ Check baseline laboratory values—BUN, creatinine, electrolytes, and liver enzymes.
■ Obtain a portable chest x-ray to rule out aspiration.
■ Continue magnesium sulfate 1 gm IV every hour by infusion pump. (Increase magnesium sulfate if reflexes are hyperactive; decrease magnesium sulfate if reflexes are absent or for oliguria.)
■ Keep calcium gluconate or calcium chloride at bedside in case of magnesium overdose (dosage is 1 gm IV push).
■ Check reflexes, urinary output, and respirations every hour. Expect a urine output of at least 30 ml/hour and respirations of 14 per minute.
■ Treat diastolic pressures of 100 or more with hydralazine, IV, in a 5-mg bolus; then with a regulated IV dose—100 mg hydralazine in 250 mg normal saline in a plastic IV bag—to maintain a diastolic pressure of 80 to 90.

Rules for delivering the eclamptic patient

1. Once magnesium sulfate and hydration are under way, evaluate maternal and fetal indications and make a decision within 4 hours. Do not wait for patient's condition to stabilize.
2. Do amniocentesis to check for meconium and surfactant.
3. If the cervix is favorable, treat with amniotomy and IV oxytocin induction.
4. Do cesarean section with general anesthesia when the fetus is severly premature (1,500 gm or less), when the cervix is unfavorable, or

when there is a breech presentation. Do not use conduction anesthesia, because of decreased blood volume.

5. For patients in labor, avoid barbiturates and narcotics that depress the fetus. Use local anesthesia or pudendal block for vaginal deliveries. Use general anesthesia for cesarean section.

REFERENCES
1. Sibai BM, Lipshitz J, Anderson GD, et al: Reassessment of intravenous $MgSO_4$ therapy in preeclampsia-eclampsia. Obstet Gynecol 57:199, 1981
2. Lewis PJ, Bulpitt CJ, Zuspan FP: A comparison of current British and American practice in the management of hypertension in pregnancy. J Obstet Gynaecol Br Commonw. In press
3. Zuspan FP, Ward MC: Improved fetal salvage in eclampsia. Obstet Gynecol 26:893, 1965
4. Pritchard JA, Stone SR: Clinical and laboratory observations on eclampsia. Am J Obstet Gynecol 99:754, 1967
5. Zuspan FP: Problems encountered in the treatment of pregnancy induced hypertension. Am J Obstet Gynecol 131:591, 1978

Mary Jo O'Sullivan, MD

Ruptured uterus: Still a challenge

14

Diagnosis should be based not only on classical signs and symptoms, but also on subtle signs of blood loss. When the rupture is recognized and treated early enough to prevent excessive blood loss and shock, maternal and fetal mortality and morbidity can usually be avoided.

If you are a practicing obstetrician, you may never encounter a case of ruptured uterus. Occurring in 0.03% to 0.08% (1:1,204 to 1:2,861) of all deliveries, it is among the rarest of obstetric emergencies (Table 14-1).[1-7] By rupture, I mean complete separation of the uterine musculature through all layers. I don't mean the dehiscence that characterizes incomplete rupture. But anyone who has seen a case will agree that the faster you confirm the diagnosis and start treatment, the better the chances of good maternal and fetal outcome.

Since cesarean section has replaced many obstetric manipulations in the uterus and eliminated prolonged dysfunctional labors, you would expect a decrease in the incidence of traumatic rupture and an increase in scar rupture. Table 14-2 classifies the deliveries listed in Table 14-1 as pre-1960 (group A) and post-1970 (group B). It shows that the distribution of ruptures among Krishna-Menon's three categories (spontaneous, traumatic, and scar) has not changed significantly over the two time periods.[8] However, when ruptures

Table 14-1. Summary of ruptured uteri studies*

Author	Total ruptures	Total patients	Incidence (%)	Total	Uterine scar Previous low segment	Uterine scar Classical cesarean	Other	Traumatic	Spontaneous
Erving[2] (1930-1956)	37	96,153	0.04	20	3	15	2	15	2
Ferguson[3] (1935-1955)	84 (42)	101,108	0.08-0.04	18	5	13	—	9	15
Ware[6] (1932-1956)	40	70,837	0.06	16	2	14	—	15	9
Donnelly[1] (1948-1961)	43	118,626	0.04	15	13	—	2	15	13
Schrinsky[5] (1950-1975)	47 (34)	126,770	0.04–0.03	12	4	8	—	10	12
Mercer[4] (1971-1979)	18 (15)	51,500	0.04–0.03	6	4	1	1	5	4
Totals	**269 (211)**	**564,994**	**0.05–0.04**	**87**	**32**	**51**	**5**	**69**	**55**
Percent of total ruptures				41.23%				32.70%	26.07%

( ) Indicates only overt ruptures. Percentages are based upon overt ruptures only.
*Adapted from O'Sullivan MJ, Fumia F, Halsinger K, et al.[11]

are considered as a percentage of total deliveries, all categories show a decrease in the period since 1970. The decreases are greatest in the scar and traumatic groups. Perhaps a change in surgical technique is responsible for the downward trend in the scar group. After 1970, most abdominal deliveries would have been low segment. Before 1960, there would have been more classical sections. And too, the trend toward more vaginal deliveries of patients who previously had cesareans may have increased the incidence of scar rupture.

Numerous classifications of uterine rupture have been proposed, based on a variety of anatomic and etiologic factors. Probably the simplest is that of Krishna-Menon.[8] Spontaneous and traumatic ruptures are usually more catastrophic than the scar variety in terms of signs, symptoms, and maternal and fetal prognosis. Scar rupture, the most common type, usually is secondary to rupture of a previous cesarean scar. The distinction between traumatic and spontaneous rupture is based on cause; spontaneous rupture is unrelated to any known predisposing factor.

Table 14-2. Distribution of ruptures by type has remained constant over several decades

Type rupture	Before 1960 Deliveries (%)	Before 1960 Ruptures (%)	After 1970 Deliveries (%)	After 1970 Ruptures (%)
Scar	0.018	42.59	0.012	40.00
Traumatic	0.014	33.33	0.009	33.33
Spontaneous	0.010	24.07	0.008	26.66

What are the causes?

Any of the following factors may cause uterine rupture—and they may be additive:

■ Trauma antecedent to the present pregnancy, including curettage; uterine perforation—either recognized or unrecognized—inflicted by a sound, curette, or similar instrument; previous uterine surgery—myomectomy; cesarean section, hysterotomy, or Strassmann or similar procedure; or cornual resection.

■ Obstetric factors in the present pregnancy, including excessive uterine stimulation—spontaneous or drug induced; operative obstetrics—version, extraction, midforceps; hydrocephalus or other obstructive fetal mass; shoulder dystocia; neglected labor; excessive fundal pressure, grand multiparity; abruptio placentae; trophoblastic disease; or placenta increta-percreta.

■ Other factors, such as uterine anomalies, trauma, cornual pregnancy, or unknown causes.

Making the diagnosis

Most ruptures occur in the lower uterine segment. Rupture of the unscarred uterus, most common during labor or delivery, is usually longitudinal in the region of the uterine vessels, and most often on the left.[9] Since the vessels are involved, often there is excessive external or concealed bleeding.

The classical symptoms are sudden tearing abdominal pain followed by relief of pain, shock, loss of fetal heart tones, cessation of contractions, tachycardia, and abdominal tenderness. But pain may be minimal. There may be some maternal restlessness, tachycardia, and retraction or ascent of the presenting part if delivery has not occurred. Fetal heart tones initially may be stable. Bleeding may be out into the broad ligament and so may remain in the retroperitoneum and concealed. These symptoms, which are not classical, contribute to delay in diagnosis. Bleeding that is intra-abdominal usually gives more obvious signs, consistent with an acute abdomen.

Since uterine contractions usually do not cease when the lower segment ruptures, spontaneous or assisted vaginal delivery may be concluded successfully. However, rupture may occur during delivery as a result of forceps injury, fundal pressure, shoulder dystocia, or difficulty with the aftercoming head. Again, bleeding may be external or concealed. And if external bleeding is attributed to concomitant cervical or vaginal lacerations, the low-segment laceration may go unrecognized until the patient has persistent unexplained bleeding and is in shock, or until she is explored for uncontrolled bleeding with the diagnosis made retrospectively.

Persistent bleeding despite a well-contracted uterus and no apparent lacerations should arouse your suspicions. In fact, you should think of the possibility of a rupture whenever a patient has any of the predisposing factors. Think rupture and you are unlikely to miss it!

A scarred uterus should alert you to the possibility of uterine rupture. Here too, rupture is more common in the lower segment and may be very subtle. The site of rupture—the scar—is relatively avascular, so bleeding is often less than in spontaneous or traumatic rupture. Should rupture occur during labor, contractions will frequently continue. Maternal tachycardia, restlessness, and change of personality may be seen. Fetal heart tones may or may not change, depending on uteroplacental/umbilical continuity. Irregularity over the suprapubic area or swelling and retraction of the presenting part are also clues. Lower abdominal tenderness and pain are common symptoms during labor and therefore may or may not be helpful in making the diagnosis. Hypotension is usually a late feature, unless the rupture extends out into the broad ligament.

While spontaneous and traumatic ruptures rarely occur except during labor, some 24% of scarred uteri may rupture before labor begins.[10] Almost invariably, fundal ruptures are found in uteri scarred by classical cesareans or myomectomies. The presenting signs and symptoms are more obvious and also classical. Occasionally, the site of rupture is occluded or compressed by a fetal part. Bleeding controlled in this way delays diagnosis. Should a fundal scar rupture during labor, continuous pain may replace the intermittent contractions of labor, followed by a tearing sensation, and then relief. Uterine contractions cease, fetal heart tones are lost, and the signs and symptoms of blood loss become obvious.

Classical cesarean sections are unusual today, although hysterotomies are still done occasionally. When you are dealing with an immigrant population, you can't always be sure a previous cesarean was low segment. Finally, the incidence of premature delivery by cesarean section has increased. Many of these incisions start out as low segment vertical but may become classical because of a poorly developed lower uterine segment. Therefore, we have to think of the possibility of rupture in cases of abdominal pain and uterine scars and to search for other signs and symptoms to confirm or rule out the diagnosis.

Once suspicion is sufficiently aroused, prepare for immediate fluid replacement; transfusion, which may be massive; and abdominal or transvaginal exploration. Maternal death is more common following traumatic (24%) and spontaneous rupture (11%) than after scar ruptures (3.07%).[11] However, much of the recent literature reports no maternal or fetal deaths.[12-14]

Managing the rupture

Patients with previous cesarean sections who are candidates for a trial of labor must fit all the selection criteria (Table 14-3), be closely monitored during labor, and have a normoprogressive labor, ideally without oxytocin

111

Table 14-3. Selection criteria for trial of labor in previous cesarean patients

- Only one previous low-segment transverse cesarean with no extension documented by operative note
- Readily available blood, anesthesia, and operating facilities on same floor as labor suite
- Previous indication no longer exists
- Clinically adequate pelvis for this baby
- No medical or obstetric complications
- Patient acceptance and understanding of risks of abdominal and vaginal delivery
- No previous uterine rupture

(although the latter is not totally contraindicated). Most properly selected patients will deliver vaginally without incident. When patients, physicians, and nurses are all tuned in to the possibility of rupture, medical personnel will intervene more often and earlier than in unscarred uteri. This will lessen blood loss and improve maternal and fetal outcomes.

After vaginal delivery of a previous cesarean patient, a careful exam is necessary to search for a uterine defect. If this exam makes you suspect a defect or asymptomatic rupture, and the abdominal cavity is not entered, you can manage conservatively, watching carefully for any evidence of vaginal or concealed bleeding. Signs of concealed hemorrhage are tachycardia (postpartum most patients develop relative bradycardia), restlessness, hypotension, increasing fundal height, or a fundus pushed to one side despite an empty bladder. Vaginal exam may disclose fullness anteriorly (again despite an empty bladder) or in either parametrial region. However, if the abdominal cavity was entered or there is evidence of bleeding or hematuria, laparotomy must be carried out. When there is suspicion of a rupture in a patient with an unscarred uterus, do a careful intrauterine exam to try to palpate the defect. Once the diagnosis of rupture is confirmed or sufficient suspicion remains, laparotomy should follow. When there is little doubt that uterine rupture has taken place, proceed to laparotomy without examining the uterus.

The treatment of choice is total abdominal hysterectomy. Occasionally, this may have to be preceded by hypogastric artery ligation to control bleeding in the broad ligament. When hemorrhage is massive, you may also find temporary aortic compression very helpful in controlling bleeding while you are trying to obtain better visualization. Repair is rarely, if ever, indicated in a ruptured, previously intact uterus, because of increased risk of rupture the second time around.[15] However, you may consider scar repair when patients desire more children. Any subsequent delivery should be carried out by cesarean section.

Uterine rupture can be associated with very high maternal and fetal mortality and morbidity unless it is recognized and treated early enough to prevent prolonged excessive blood loss and shock secondary to uterine vessel involvement. The diagnosis should be based not only on classical signs and symptoms, but also on subtle signs of blood loss.

REFERENCES

1. Donnelly JP, Franzoni KF: Uterine rupture. A thirty year survey. Obstet Gynecol 23:774, 1964
2. Erving HW: Rupture of the uterus. Am J Obstet Gynecol 71:251, 1957
3. Ferguson RK, Reid DK: Rupture of the uterus: A twenty year report. Am J Obstet Gynecol 76:172, 1958
4. Mercer CA: *Uterine rupture during pregnancy. Annual Obstetric Gynecologic Resident's Day Symposium.* Emory University, Atlanta, June 1980
5. Schrinsky DC, Benson R: Rupture of the pregnant uterus: A review. Obstet Gynecol Surv 33:217, 1978
6. Ware HH, Jarrett AQ, Reda FA: Rupture of the gravid uterus. Am J Obstet Gynecol 76:181, 1958
7. Golan A, Sandbank O, Rubin A: Rupture of the pregnant uterus. Obstet Gynecol 56:549, 1981
8. Krishna-Menon MD: Rupture of the uterus: A review of 164 cases. J Obstet Gynaecol Br Commonw 69:18, 1962
9. Voogd LB, Wood HH, Powell DV: Ruptured uterus. Obstet Gynecol 7:70, 1956
10. Eames HH: A study of the management of pregnancies subsequent to cesarean section. Am J Obstet Gynecol 65:944, 1953
11. O'Sullivan MJ, Fumia F, Holsinger K, et al: Vaginal delivery after cesarean section. Clin Perinatol 8:131, 1981
12. Garnet JD: Uterine rupture during pregnancy. An analysis of 133 patients. Obstet Gynecol 23:898, 1964
13. Gibbs CE: Planned vaginal delivery following cesarean section. Clin Obstet Gynecol 23:507, 1980
14. McGarry JA: The management of patients previously delivered by cesarean section. J Obstet Gynaecol Br Commonw 76:137, 1969
15. Weingold AB: Rupture of the gravid uterus. Surg Gynecol Obstet 122:1233, 1966

John W. Scanlon, MD

Fast action for the distressed newborn

Babies born with breathing difficulties need speedy, expert resuscitation. Delivery rooms should be prepared and equipped to deal with acute perinatal asphyxia, shock, meconium aspiration, and hydrops fetalis.

Conditions that interrupt the placenta's capacity for supplying oxygen and removing carbon dioxide and hydrogen ions can cause fetal hypoxemia, hypercapnia, or acidosis. Biochemically, this is perinatal asphyxia. Placental insufficiency may be chronic if the mother has severe hypertension, subacute with toxemia, or acute with abruption.

Perinatal asphyxia

Breathing difficulties can also begin at birth if, for example, maternally administered anesthetics diminish the neonate's respiration. Perinatal asphyxia is serious by itself and can aggravate kernicterus, necrotizing enterocolitis, or encephalopathy.

Whatever the cause of the asphyxia, the baby's homeostasis is violently altered as it attempts to maintain perfusion of the heart and central nervous system. The major goals when resuscitating an asphyxiated baby are removing carbon dioxide by establishing adequate ventilation, oxygenating tissues by raising PaO_2, and decreasing intracellular hydrogen ion (pH) concentration.

A number of excellent reviews deal with management of the acutely asphyxiated neonate.[1-5] What follows is based on our experi-

Table 15-1. Basic equipment for resuscitation

Laryngoscope with 0 or 1 Miller blades
Straight endotracheal tubes
Infant stethoscope
Overhead heating unit
Bulb syringe
Sideport suction catheters (5 to 10 French)
Doppler flow probe and newborn sphygmomanometer
Umbilical venous catheter set
Butterfly needles (23 and 25 gauge)
Neonatal intracatheters (23 and 25 gauge)
Sodium bicarbonate (neonatal dilution)
Albumin (25%)
Dextrose (5% in water)
Epinephrine (1:10,000 dilution)

ence at Columbia Hospital for Women, Washington, D.C.[6]

Equipment. The equipment needed for neonatal resuscitation is not extensive (Table 15-1), but must be in perfect working order. Before each resuscitation, check the laryngoscope bulb and battery, heaters, face masks, endotracheal tubes, and suction and oxygen systems. We install an 80-ml mucus trap in line to gather a gastric or tracheal specimen during resuscitation. Later, if needed, this material may be analyzed for surfactant content, neutrophil count, and fetal and maternal blood.

Delivery room personnel should be assigned to collect basic patient data, and one person should be responsible for recording all resuscitative efforts (see Figure 15-1).

Procedures. Aspirate the oropharynx with a bulb syringe as soon as the head is expelled. A DeLee trap is mandatory when amniotic fluid is meconium stained. Obtain a doubly clamped segment of umbilical cord for blood gas measurements to document extent of intrauterine asphyxia. This step is clinically and medicolegally important.

Whoever takes the infant from the obstetrician should be gowned but need not wear gloves. The infant is received in a warm, absorbent blanket, transferred immediately to a warming table, and placed in a head-down position, with a blanket roll under the shoulders to extend the neck slightly. If the infant's head is turned to one side, secretions will be easier to remove because they will accumulate in the corner of the mouth. The optimal time for cord clamping has not been determined.

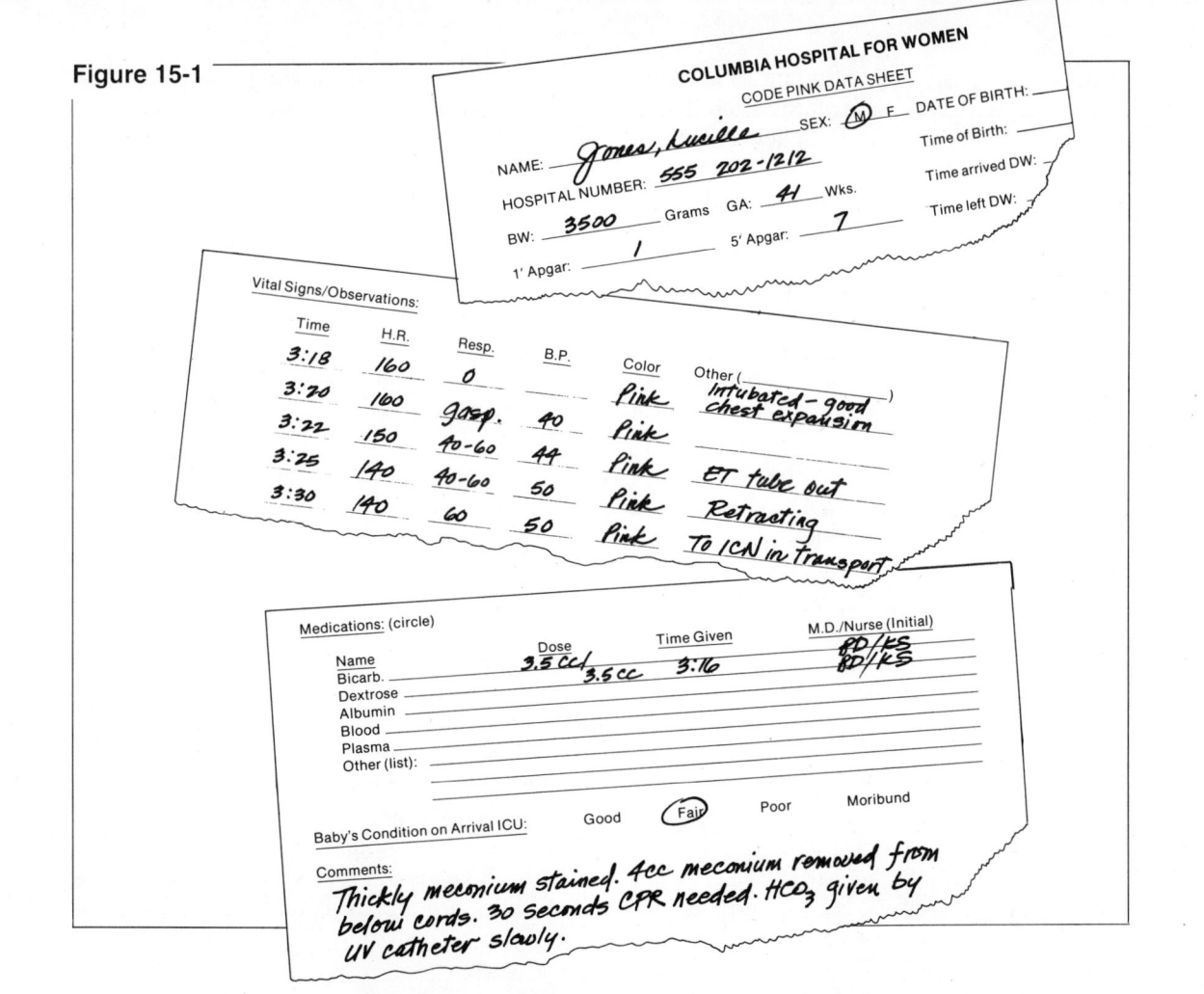

Figure 15-1

COLUMBIA HOSPITAL FOR WOMEN
CODE PINK DATA SHEET

NAME: Jones, Lucille SEX: (M) F DATE OF BIRTH: _____
HOSPITAL NUMBER: 555 202-1212 Time of Birth: _____
BW: 3500 Grams GA: 41 Wks. Time arrived DW: _____
1' Apgar: 1   5' Apgar: 7 Time left DW: _____

Vital Signs/Observations:

Time	H.R.	Resp.	B.P.	Color	Other
3:18	160	0		Pink	Intubated - good chest expansion
3:20	100	gasp.	40	Pink	
3:22	150	40-60	44	Pink	ET tube out
3:25	140	40-60	50	Pink	Retracting
3:30	140	60	50	Pink	To ICN in transport

Medications: (circle)

Name	Dose	Time Given	M.D./Nurse (Initial)
Bicarb.	3.5 cc		PD/KS
Dextrose	3.5 cc	3:16	PD/KS
Albumin			
Blood			
Plasma			
Other (list):			

Baby's Condition on Arrival ICU: Good   (Fair)   Poor   Moribund

Comments: Thickly meconium stained. 4cc meconium removed from below cords. 30 seconds CPR needed. HCO₃ given by UV catheter slowly.

117

Transfer of an asphyxiated infant to an experienced resuscitator, therefore, should take precedence over arbitrary policy about the time of cord clamping.

All delivery room personnel should be familiar with the Apgar scoring system, which is simply a measure of neonatal vital and primitive neurologic capacity. The Apgar scores should be ascertained immediately and serially during resuscitation.[7,8] If the Apgar score is 8 or above, keeping the baby warm may be all that is necessary. After a high-risk delivery, however, the baby must not be dismissed from care just because 1- and 5-minute Apgar scores are normal. Such a baby must be watched until it seems clear that problems are unlikely.

If the baby is mildly depressed (Apgar of 5 to 7), it may need only 100% oxygen by free-flow mask or general stimulation. Usually, positive pressure ventilation (PPV) is unnecessary because such infants are breathing spontaneously.

Some positive pressure ventilators must be pumped. Just holding such a device across the airway without rhythmically squeezing the bag will asphyxiate the baby. We strongly recommend having two oxygen delivery systems in each resuscitation area: one attached to the manual ventilator, the other to a free-flow delivery system. Don't use blast insufflation pressures.

When a baby is moderately depressed (Apgar of 3 or 4), provide 100% oxygen by intermittent PPV, initially by bag and mask. If bradycardia—FHR under 100 beats per minute (bpm)—does not promptly reverse with PPV, begin intermittent mechanical ventilation using an endotracheal tube.

We find 100% oxygen beneficial for asphyxia, because a rising arterial Po_2 is the major determinant of adequate neonatal pulmonary blood flow. Exposing an asphyxiated baby briefly to 100% oxygen does not increase the risk of oxygen toxicity.

The most important indication of adequate ventilation is that the baby's chest wall should move with each breath during mechanical ventilation. If it does not, you should determine whether the airway is clogged, the trachea obstructed, your technique poor, or your equipment broken. The problem must be corrected immediately.

The severely compromised neonate (Apgar of 1 to 2) needs aggressive resuscitation, initially with bag and mask and then by endotracheal ventilation with 100% oxygen. If the pulse is persistently below 100 bpm (or below 60 at any time), closed-chest cardiac massage must be done. Two skilled resuscitators must be present, one for ventilation and one for cardiac massage. This is performed by placing two fingers in the middle of the infant's sternum and compressing this halfway to the spinal column (cycled rates between 60 and 80 times per minute are optimal).

If closed-chest massage is not effective, try intracardiac epinephrine (0.1 mg diluted to 1 ml). To administer, I insert a 21-gauge needle below the costal margin to the left of the xiphoid, angling the needle upward and slightly towards the midline. Dark ventricular blood wells into the syringe when the needle enters the ventricle.

If cardiac massage is necessary, assume severe metabolic acidosis. Administer dilute sodium bicarbonate (2 mEq/kg estimated weight) slowly into the umbilical vein. Bicarbonate, epinephrine, and colloids are the main medications used in the delivery room. The prime emphasis in newborn resuscitation should be reversing cardiorespiratory dysfunction, providing adequate ventilation, and ensuring thermal homeostasis.

Keeping the baby warm is especially important. Proper drying and wrapping at the time of birth will preserve the infant's thermal environment and an overhead radiant warmer will reduce heat loss. Unfortunately, vigorous resuscitative efforts frequently block the output from the overhead warmer. Therefore, make sure the infant is dry and expose only the part of the body necessary for observation or hands-on care.

For adequate resuscitation and stabilization, the baby's peripheral vascular perfusion must be maintained. Capillary filling time is a useful measure of cutaneous blood flow. Press on the infant's skin and see how long it takes for the blanched area to resume its previous color. Normally, this should take only 3 to 4 seconds.

Blood pressure measurements taken with a Doppler pulse flow detector are also valuable. Apply the pressure cuff above the pulse to be measured and lower pressure until you hear the pulse. This value approximates the systolic blood pressure, which you can compare with norms for various birthweights.[9]

Practical guides for artificial mechanical ventilation and endotracheal tube insertion are available,[1,2,4] but there is no substitute for direct training, using dummies and live newborn animals, and periodic review of the procedures.[10] Personnel who rarely perform resuscitations may be unsure of invasive techniques, even with periodic review. This is particularly true of endotracheal intubation, which may be risky for the inexperienced to do. Bag and mask techniques can provide excellent oxygenation and ventilation for a relatively long time. Remember, chest movement is the hallmark of adequate ventilation and a pulse rate over 100 bpm suggests oxygenation at least of myocardial tissue. The long-term neurologic outcome for even severely asphyxiated neonates is surprisingly good, although the onset of symptoms such as seizures, hypotonia, or hypertonia in the immediate neonatal period is worrisome.[11]

Cardiovascular collapse

The baby's intravascular volume must be expanded to maintain tissue perfusion when there is acute blood loss or asphyxial shock. Shock from blood loss may occur with vasa previa and also in fetomaternal or fetofetal transfusions. The pathophysiology of hypotension with low peripheral perfusion includes asphyxia.

The neurovascular response to asphyxia is to maintain myocardial and CNS perfusion by reducing blood flow to the peripheral vessels. The umbilical vessels are under limited sympathetic control. During asphyxia, there is relatively more blood than normal in the placenta. Following birth, and after acidosis has been corrected, the neonate's blood volume may be insufficient when the peripheral vessels fill. The infant will be pale, blood pressure may be substantially lowered, and capillary filling time may be prolonged. Immediate volume replacement is necessary.

When there is a high risk of neonatal shock—if an Apt test has revealed fetal hemoglobin or if the baby is delivered before 30 weeks' gestation—have Rh-negative blood available that has been cross-matched with the mother's. For acute cases, the dose is 10 ml fresh blood/kg estimated birthweight. If blood is not available give salt-poor albumin, 1 gm/kg estimated birthweight as a 5% solution. If the baby has lost blood and no maternally cross-matched blood is available, use heparinized blood from the placenta. The dose of heparin is 1 unit/ml blood drawn.

Intrauterine asphyxia severe enough to produce myocardial ischemia with congestive heart failure may cause systemic hypotension and peripheral hypoperfusion. In these cases, volume expansion is not beneficial, but measures to control congestive heart failure and the administration of a positive inotropic agent (isoproterenol) may be. Infants in this type of shock will have hepatomegaly, a myocardial ischemic pattern on ECG, and the ubiquitous association of hypoglycemia. The blood sugar can be checked with a reagent strip (Dextrostix). Because diagnosis is difficult in the delivery room, assume that neonatal shock is hypovolemic and treat immediately by volume expansion.

Meconium aspiration

Whenever there is meconium in the amniotic fluid, have a skilled neonatal resuscitator present at delivery, because the newborn may be asphyxiated. More important, aspiration of meconium can start a downward spiral of pneumonia, ventilatory insufficiency, hypoxemia, acidosis, brain damage, and death. Gregory and co-workers showed that PPV or respiratory stimulation at birth will impel meconium into the lung's periphery.[12] This thick, viscid material must be removed before the infant's first breath. Furthermore, almost 10% of infants with meconium in their airways have none in their mouths or oropharynges. If every baby with thick meconium-stained amniotic fluid had direct laryngoscopy and tracheal suction, death and morbidity from the meconium-aspiration syndrome would be reduced almost to zero.

To remove the meconium, carefully suction the oropharynx with a DeLee catheter as soon as the head is free. After completing delivery, pass the infant promptly to the resuscitator, who can examine the trachea with a laryngoscope. Any tracheal meconium should be removed by direct suction using a large-bore (10 to 12 French) catheter, which usually requires at least 100 cm H_2O pressure. Occasionally, if there are large chunks of meconium, direct laryngoscopy with the use of a large-bore endotracheal tube and mouth-to-tube suction may be necessary.

Hydrops fetalis

Fluid accumulation resulting from Rh disease is becoming rare, but hydrops from other causes still occurs. The fatality rate approaches 100%, yet affected infants, if properly managed, can survive with an excellent prognosis.[13,14]

Careful, expert ventilatory control is the first step in caring for the hydropic baby. Two people skilled in resuscitation are needed in the delivery room: one to intubate and manage the ventilation, the other to maintain tissue perfusion and adequate colloid oncotic pressure as the extensive anasarca is decreased. Be sure 100 ml of maternally cross-matched Rh-negative blood is available in the delivery room whenever there is even a hint that a hydropic infant is to be delivered. The person responsible for maintaining perfusion should catheterize the umbilical vein and perform an abdominal paracentesis. As blood is transfused into the vein in 10-ml aliquots, an equal volume of abdominal ascitic fluid is removed through a #22 intracatheter inserted in the left peritoneal gut or through a 22-gauge butterfly needle placed in a more anterior abdominal location.

Because the major pathophysiologic deficit in hydrops fetalis is low serum protein,[15] simultaneously removing ascitic fluid and replacing blood in isovolumetric amounts maintains adequate tissue oxygenation and colloid oncotic pressure. The procedure, however, must be done carefully: removing ascitic fluid too rapidly may precipitate shock and infusing blood too quickly may aggravate congestive heart failure. When sufficient fluid is removed to allow adequate pulmonary ventilation, the baby can be transferred to the NICU for an immediate exchange transfusion. A diligent search for the etiology of hydrops is essential. Take a blood sample before the transfusion, and examine the placenta, because vascular anomalies can produce hydrops.

What to tell the mother

The senior member of the neonatal team should succinctly but compassionately tell the mother what has been done and what the prognosis is. If possible, let her see the baby in the transport incubator. Show her where the NICU is located and tell her which physicians and nurses will care for her baby. Inform her if transfer to a tertiary center is contemplated. Such communication is an integral part of resuscitative procedure.

In summary, the techniques of neonatal resuscitation are simple and straightfoward. The keys to success are an obstetrician who anticipates all potential problems and other personnel in the delivery room ready to begin resuscitative efforts promptly and continue them until the baby can breathe on its own.

REFERENCES

1. Akamatsu TJ: Management of the newborn, including resuscitation. Clin Obstet Gynecol 2:673, 1975
2. Fisher DE, Paton JB: Resuscitation of the newborn infant. In Klaus MH, Fanaroff AA (eds): *Care of the High-Risk Neonate.* ed 2. Philadelphia: Saunders, 1979
3. Gluck L (ed): *Intrauterine Asphyxia and the Developing Brain.* Chicago: Year Book Medical Publishers, 1977
4. Gregory GA: Cardio-pulmonary resuscitation of the newborn. In Shnider SM, Moya FP (eds): *The Anesthesiologist, Mother and Newborn.* Baltimore: Williams & Wilkins, 1974
5. Volpe JJ: Perinatal-hypoxic ischemic brain injury, Pediatr Clin North Am 23:383, 1976
6. Daze AM, Scanlon JW: *Code Pink: A System of Neonatal Resuscitation.* Baltimore: University Park Press, 1981
7. Apgar VA: Proposal for a new method of evaluation in the infant. Curr Res Anesth Analg 32:260, 1953
8. Scanlon JW: How is the baby: The Apgar score revisited. Clin Pediatr 12:61, 1973
9. Scanlon JW, Nelson T, Grylack LJ, et al: *A System of Newborn Physical Examination.* Baltimore: University Park Press, 1979
10. Harkavy KL: Learning the technical skills for resuscitation. In Daze AM, Scanlon JW (eds): *Code Pink: A System of Neonatal Resuscitation.* Baltimore: University Park Press, 1981
11. Grylack LJ: The outcome for asphyxiated babies. In Daze AM, Scanlon JW (eds): *Code Pink: A System of Neonatal Resuscitation.* Baltimore: University Park Press, 1981
12. Gregory GA, Goodings C, Phibbs RH, et al: Meconium aspiration in infants: A prospective study. J Pediatr 85:848, 1974
13. Oh W, Arbit J, Blonsky ER, et al: Neurologic and psychometric follow-up study of erythroblastotic infants requiring intrauterine transfusions. Obstet Gynecol 100:330, 1971
14. Scanlon JW, Muirhead DM: Hydrops fetalis due to anti-Kell isoimmune disease: Survival with longterm outcome. J Pediatr 88:484, 1976
15. Phibbs RH, Johnson R, Tooley WH: Cardiorespiratory status of erythroblastotic newborn infants. Pediatrics 53:13, 1974

Philip B. Mead, MD

Postpartum endometritis

16

Once a working diagnosis is made, choice of antimicrobial therapy depends on susceptibility patterns in your hospital and degree of severity.

Inadequately treated, postpartum endometritis may progress to endomyometritis, pelvic cellulitis, pelvic abscess, or septic pelvic thrombophlebitis. Early symptoms include a fever greater than 100.4°F and uterine tenderness, with or without foul lochia. The uterus is often subinvoluted.

The U.S. Joint Committee on Maternal Welfare's definition of standard puerperal morbidity—a temperature of 100.4°F in any two of the first 10 days postpartum, exclusive of the first 24 hours—probably is no longer useful in the modern hospital setting. Because patients are being discharged earlier now, these criteria can no longer be fully applied. Moreover, many patients with infection respond to antibiotic therapy so rapidly that they do not meet the temperature requirements for standard morbidity.

Predisposing factors

Incidence is overwhelmingly related to the route of delivery. Following vaginal delivery, incidences range from 0.9% to 3.9%; the higher rates are found on services caring for indigent patients. Following cesarean section, the incidence on most private services is about 10%; it is as high as 50% or more on large teaching services caring for indigent patients.

Although prolonged membrane rupture, midforceps delivery, anemia, and maternal soft-tissue trauma are commonly mentioned as predisposing factors following vaginal delivery, these events—not identified in most patients who develop infections—are probably *relative* risk factors. Predisposing factors following cesarean section include duration of rupture of membranes and labor, duration of internal fetal monitoring, antepartum or postpartum anemia, number of vaginal examinations, obesity, and presence of meconium. Sophisticated statistical procedures like discriminate or regression analysis have failed to settle the question of which of these events relate most directly to subsequent endometritis. In general, patients undergoing elective repeat sections or primary sections before onset of labor and membrane rupture are at low risk of developing postpartum endometritis, whereas patients undergoing cesarean following prolonged labor, prolonged rupture of membranes, or prolonged internal fetal monitoring are at high risk.

Responsible organisms

Organisms normally found in the vaginal flora are the usual causes of endometritis. They include gram-negative aerobic bacilli (*Escherichia coli* most commonly, but occasionally *Klebsiella* species, *Enterobacter* species, or *Proteus mirabilis*); anaerobic bacteria (especially peptostreptococci, but occasionally *Bacteroides fragilis* and other anaerobes); and enterococci (*Streptococcus fecalis*). Group B β-hemolytic streptococcal endometritis occurs infrequently and is often self-limited, although severe infections, including meningitis, and death have been reported. Group A β-hemolytic streptococcal endometritis, the dreaded "childbed fever" of Semmelweis and Oliver Wendell Holmes, is fortunately rare. Its onset is often florid and the lochia is usually not foul. *Clostridium perfringens*, a rare cause of puerperal infection, produces a characteristic clinical picture. In severe cases, massive intravascular hemolysis causes jaundice, mahogany-colored urine, and extreme degrees of anemia in an incredibly short time—within hours. Such hemolysis frequently results in acute renal failure secondary to lower nephron nephrosis. *Clostridium tetani* endometritis is rare, with fewer than 150 cases reported. Mortality is high, however.

Platt reports that the commonest cause of postpartum fever following vaginal delivery at Boston City Hospital is *Mycoplasma hominis* infection, defined by a fourfold or greater rise in mycoplasmacidal antibody titer.[1] The clinical significance of this finding is unclear since most of these patients did not have physical findings compatible with endometritis.

Difficulty of obtaining meaningful culture specimens is a stumbling block in the precise bacteriologic evaluation of the patient with endometritis. Although numerous transcervical techniques have been tried,[2] no practical way has been found to obtain uncontaminated endometrial cultures. Gibbs and O'Dell, using a transcervical culture technique designed to avoid contamination, found no difference between the bacterial flora of the endometrial cavity in patients with endometritis and those who were not infected.[3] Transabdominal needle aspiration of the endometrial cavity avoids the problem of lower tract contamination, but is not a practical approach in routine patient care. Blood cultures can be helpful, but are positive in fewer than 1% of patients delivered vaginally, and in fewer than 5% of those delivered by section.

Making the diagnosis

Remember that postpartum endometritis is a rare occurrence following vaginal delivery in a nonindigent patient. Accordingly, assiduously rule out other causes of fever in such patients before accepting postpartum endometritis as the entity to be treated. Failure to heed this warning occasionally results in delayed and inappropriate treatment of other, potentially life-threatening disorders.

The differential diagnosis of postpartum endometritis includes urinary tract infection, mastitis, appendicitis, subgluteal or retropsoas synergistic bacterial infection, infectious mononucleosis or other viral disease, septic pelvic thrombophlebitis, and right ovarian vein syndrome.

Obtaining cultures

Once a working diagnosis of postpartum endometritis has been made, do a pelvic examination on an appropriate examining table. Using a sterile speculum, visualize the cervix, swab it with povidone-iodine, and take a transcervical swab for aerobic culture. If the culture report shows group A β-hemolytic streptococci, you can assume that this is the responsible pathogen, as it is never part of the normal vaginal flora. This finding has major epidemiologic as well as therapeutic implications. If group B β-hemolytic streptococci are isolated, they may or may not be the cause, as these organisms are found in as many as 35% of normal gravidas. However, the presence of group B streptococci from the vagina has obvious neonatal implications. The finding of *Clostridium perfringens* in the absence of the typical clostridial syndrome probably suggests that the organism represents only normal flora (*Clostridium perfringens* is found in the vaginal flora of approximately 5% of normal patients). A heavy growth or pure culture of *Clostridium perfringens* should alert you to explore further. With these exceptions, isolation of other bacteria is not helpful, since it is impossible to differentiate between infection and contamination with normal flora. We therefore do not obtain anaerobic cultures.

In patients who delivered vaginally, you can gently insert an empty sponge forceps into the uterine cavity when you do the speculum exam for aerobic culture. This procedure will occasionally break up a "lochial block," establishing free drainage, and will itself lyse the fever. Most obstetricians prefer not to perform this procedure after cesarean section, for fear of disrupting the uterine incision.

If the patient is initially moderately to severely ill, or if she has failed to respond to presumably appropriate therapy, it is worthwhile to obtain both aerobic and anaerobic blood cultures. Obtain additional cultures, up to a total of three sets, coincident with fever spikes.

Antimicrobial therapy

For patients with mild endometritis, antimicrobial therapy depends to some extent on susceptibility patterns of the common gram-negative aerobic bacilli in your hospital. In general, we have chosen to treat patients with mild postpartum endometritis with ampicillin (Amcill-S, Polycillin-N), 2 gm by intermittent IV administration (Soluset) initially, followed by 1.5 gm by IV Soluset every 4 hours; or cefoxitin (Mefoxin), 1 gm by IV Soluset every 4 hours. Continue therapy until the patient has been afebrile and without significant uterine tenderness for approximately three days.

The value of discharging the patient on an additional course of oral antibiotics to complete a seven- to 10-day course has never been scientifically documented. The rare patient with group A β-hemolytic streptococcal infection should, however, be treated for a total of 10 days.

It is difficult to distinguish patients with mild infections from those whose infections are severe. However, most experienced clinicians are able to make this useful distinction, based on patterns of pulse and fever, general systemic toxicity, and clinical course. If patients appear to have severe endometritis or endometritis associated with possible pelvic abscess or septic pelvic thrombophlebitis, the question is whether to cover for *Bacteroides fragilis*. While most studies find that only 15% to 20% of patients with postcesarean endometritis require such coverage for cure, including such coverage in the antibiotic regimen decreases initial therapeutic failures from 36% down to 14% or less. Moreover, review of the recent literature suggests that pelvic abscess and septic pelvic thrombophlebitis did not develop when patients were given an initial regimen effective against *B. fragilis*, whereas 7% of patients who were not on such a regimen developed one or both of these serious complications, and wound abscesses occurred twice as often.

Based on this experience, we treat patients with severe postpartum endometritis (or those suspected of having associated septic pelvic thrombophlebitis or pelvic abscess) with a regimen of clindamycin (Cleocin), 600 mg by IV Soluset every 6 hours, and tobramycin (Nebcin), 1.0 to 1.5 mg/kg IV every 8 hours. Clindamycin covers all anaerobes, including *B. fragilis*, and tobramycin covers most gram-negative aerobic bacilli. This regimen does not cover enterococci.

Patients receiving clindamycin, as well as other antibiotics, should be monitored closely for the development of diarrhea. Discontinue clindamycin when the patient has five or more stools per day. Usually, discontinuing the antibiotic is all that is necessary to treat either the diarrheal syndrome or the syndrome of pseudomembranous enterocolitis. Serious cases of pseudomembranous enterocolitis can be effectively managed with oral vancomycin (Vancocin) or oral bacitracin (Cortisporin, Neosporin, Polysporin).

Before starting aminoglycoside antibiotics such as tobramycin or gentamicin (Garamycin), take a careful history and do appropriate laboratory studies. If you find any renal compromise, or if the patient is seriously ill, it is extremely important to test serum aminoglycoside levels to ensure that toxic levels have not developed and that optimal therapeutic levels are being achieved. Draw peak-and-trough aminoglycoside levels only after the first three to five doses have been given, as it takes the drug this long to equilibrate. Obtain peak levels either 1 hour after an IM dose, or from the opposite arm as soon as an IV dose has run in. Obtain trough levels just before the next dose. Peak levels of tobramycin or gentamicin should be 4 to 10 µg/ml, and trough levels less than 2 µg/ml. Obtain a serum creatinine every other day during therapy. Other antibiotics effective against *Bacteroides fragilis* include chloramphenicol (Chloromycetin), carbenicillin (Geopen), metronidazole (Flagyl), and cefoxitin.

If fever persists, the failure of apparently appropriate antibiotic therapy can often be ascribed to failure to diagnose a pelvic or wound abscess. Search diligently for a hidden abscess by bimanual examination and examination of the abdominal wound. If you strongly suspect an abscess but cannot find it by physical examination, turn to ultrasonography, computed axial tomography (CAT), or gallium-67 scanning.

If there are no localizing signs or symptoms, begin with a gallium scan to try to identify and locate the general anatomic position of the abscess. CAT scanning or ultrasound is the most precise way to locate and characterize the mass. Once you have located the abscess, you are ready to decide on the best technique for draining it.

Patients who remain febrile, with hectic fever spikes and plateau tachycardia, even though an abscess has been ruled out, may have septic pelvic thrombophlebitis. This clinical picture, associated with an arterial oxygen below 80 mm Hg in the nonsmoker, is strongly suggestive, although this is primarily a diagnosis of exclusion. If the diagnosis is correct, full IV heparin anticoagulation will result in a rapid lysis of the fever, usually within 48 hours. Most infectious disease experts recommend instituting or continuing antimicrobial therapy, including coverage for *Bacteroides fragilis*.

A variant of septic pelvic thrombophlebitis is the so-called puerperal ovarian vein syndrome, a condition usually characterized by lower abdominal pain, fever, and a typical right paraumbilical abdominal mass. Brown and Munsick have provided an excellent review of this condition.[4] Treatment is the same for both conditions.

Epidemiology

The isolation of group A β-hemolytic streptococci from a patient with postpartum endometritis is potentially significant. This is usually a sporadic case, but serious epidemics of group A streptococcal puerperal sepsis do occur even in this era of effective antibiotics.

The rapidity with which such an epidemic can develop demands unusual vigilance.

When group A β-hemolytic streptococci are isolated from a patient with postpartum endometritis, all patients with clinical diagnosis of endometritis should have lochial cultures taken for group A streptococci. (Many services take such cultures routinely.) If a second patient is found with a positive culture, be concerned about a possible epidemic. Take the following steps: Notify local health authorities; employ strict isolation of all infected patients; institute a cohort nursery system; culture all professional and support hospital staff and relieve from duty any who are colonized; culture all newborns for group A streptococci; reduce numbers of visitors; stress adherence to aseptic technique, especially handwashing; save positive group A streptococcal cultures (for specific serotyping).

REFERENCES
1. Platt R, Lin JL, Warren JW, et al: Infection with *Mycoplasma hominis* in postpartum fever. Lancet 2:1217, 1980
2. Knuppel RA, Scerbo JC, Dzink J, et al: Quantitative transcervical uterine cultures with a new device. Obstet Gynecol 57:243, 1981
3. Gibbs RS, O'Dell TN, MacGregor RR, et al: Puerperal endometritis. A prospective microbiologic study. Am J Obstet Gynecol 121:919, 1975
4. Brown TK, Munsick RA: Puerperal ovarian vein thrombophlebitis: A syndrome. Am J Obstet Gynecol 109:263, 1971

SUGGESTED READING
Biello DR, Levitt RG, Melson GL: The roles of gallium-67 scintigraphy, ultrasonography, and computed tomography in the detection of abdominal abscess. Semin Nucl Med 9(1):58, 1979
Collins CG, Ayers WB: Suppurative pelvic thrombophlebitis. III. Surgical technique. Surgery 30:319, 1951
Cunningham FG, Hauth JC, Strong JD, et al: Infectious morbidity following cesarean section. Comparison of two treatment regimens. Obstet Gynecol 52:656, 1978
DiZerega G. Yonekura L. Roy S, et al: A comparison of clindamycin-gentamicin and penicillin-gentamicin in the treatment of post-cesarean section endomyometritis. Am J Obstet Gynecol 134:238, 1979
Gibbs RS, Jones PM, Wilder CJ: Antibiotic therapy of endometritis following cesarean section: Treatment successes and failures. Obstet Gynecol 52:31, 1978
Gibbs RS, Rodgers PJ. Castaneda YS, et al: Endometritis following vaginal delivery. Obstet Gynecol 56:555, 1980
Gibbs, RS, Weinstein AJ: Pueperal infection in the antibiotic era. Obstet Gynecol 124:769, 1976
Josey WE, Cook CC: Septic pelvic thrombophlebitis: Report of 17 patients treated with heparin. Obstet Gynecol 35:891, 1970
Ledger WJ,Gee CL, Pollin PA, et al: A new approach to patients with suspected anaerobic postpartum pelvic infections. Transabdominal uterine aspiration for culture and metronidazole for treatment. Am J Obstet Gynecol 126:1, 1976
Mariona FG, Ismail MA: *Clostridium perfringens* septicemia following cesarean section. Obstet Gynecol 56:518, 1980
Monif GRG, Hempling RE: Antibiotic therapy for the *Bacteroidaceae* in post-cesarean section infections. Obstet Gynecol 57:177, 1981
Rehu M, Nilsson CG: Risk factors for febrile morbidity associated with cesarean section. Obstet Gynecol 56:269, 1980
Sweet RL, Ledger WJ: Puerperal infectious morbidity: A two-year review. Am J Obstet Gynecol 117:1093, 1973

Editor: Ralph M. Richart, MD Conference participants: John L. Antunes, MD, Bruce A. Barron, MD, PhD, Mieczyslaw Finster, MD, Roy H. Petrie, MD, and Raymond Vande Wiele, MD.

Problem-patient conference: Subarachnoid hemorrhage in pregnancy

17

Craniotomy before delivery would expose the fetus to induction of hypotension. Terminating the pregnancy before neurosurgical intervention would expose the mother to the risk of another hemorrhage. The panel discusses the choices facing the obstetricians, neurosurgeons, and anesthesiologists in two cases.

FINSTER: In our discussion of subarachnoid hemorrhage during pregnancy, Dr. Petrie will describe two patients treated in this institution—one having a leaking cerebral aneurysm; the other, an arteriovenous malformation (AVM). Dr. Antunes will give a neurosurgeon's view of these two conditions in pregnancy. I will say a few words about the choice of anesthesia for delivery. Then Dr. Petrie and I will discuss the therapeutic dilemmas we faced, particularly concerning the patient with the aneurysm.

Patient 1: a cerebral aneurysm

PETRIE: The first patient came to Sloane Hospital for Women on November 30, 1978. She was an 18-year-old gravida 1, para 0, with an expected date of confinement on July 3,

133

1979. When seen in the screening clinic, her uterus was of approximately 10 weeks' size.

The patient was next seen in the antepartum clinic for a workup on January 9, 1979. She was an unmarried Hispanic with a family background of medical problems. She had had a herniorrhaphy as a child and excision of lipomas. A maternal aunt had had a twin gestation; her grandfather had diabetes mellitus; and another grandfather died of cancer. Her laboratory values included the following: a positive immunoassay for pregnancy; a negative serologic test for lues; blood type, A Rh positive; hematocrit, 35%; a negative voided urinalysis with 1+ bacteria (culture and sensitivity revealed more than 10,000 *Staphylococcus epidermidis);* Pap smear, class I; rubella titer, 1:64.

On physical examination, her uterus was three finger-breadths under the umbilicus. She was 56 inches tall, weighed 98 pounds, and had a blood pressure of 120/70 mm Hg. It was noted that quickening had occurred a day before her visit in the clinic.

The patient was given multivitamins [Natalins] and advised to return in a month. But she did not return until April 25, 1979—when the uterus was of approximately 32 weeks' size—complaining of severe headache, frontal in nature and radiating through the back of the neck. Nausea, vomiting, a stiff neck with nuchal rigidity, and photophobia were also present. The gynecologist asked for a neurologic consultation. Because of the pain, meperidine [Demerol] was administered. A lumbar puncture was accomplished with an opening pressure of 120 mm Hg of CSF. There was bloody fluid without clearing, and moderate xanthochromia. The diagnosis was that of subdural hemorrhage.

The patient was admitted to the Neurological Institute and given betamethasone to induce pulmonary maturity [in the manner of G.C. Liggins, National Women's Hospital, Auckland]. A CAT scan revealed an increased density, probably fresh blood, at the base of the septum. It was felt this was a subarachnoid hemorrhage from a leaking aneurysm. The patient was given aminocaproic acid [Amicar], phenobarbital, meperidine, prochlorperazine [Compazine], and hydralazine hydrochloride [Apresoline]. When angiography was performed on April 27, the aneurysm ruptured, and dye extravasated into the adjacent tissue. The surgeons, who described it as a posterior-inferior cerebral artery aneurysm, felt it could be clipped only after the patient was medically stable. Ultrasound determinations indicated a fetal biparietal diameter of 8.2 cm, consistent with a gestation of 33 weeks.

On May 3, her neck was still stiff, with occasional diplopia, and her right eye was occluded. On May 11, a CAT scan showed the hemorrhage had subsided; on May 22, she was less lethargic, better oriented, and had a stable blood pressure.

On May 24, in the Neurological Institute, a low flap elliptical cesarean section was performed, under lumbar epidural anesthesia, delivering a 2,020-gm female with Apgar scores of 7, 9, and 9 at 1, 2, and 5 minutes. The blood loss was estimated at 600 ml. Then the craniotomy was performed, by a Pool incision [J. Lawrence Pool, a pioneer in aneurysm surgery]. The arteries were isolated and the aneurysm was clipped after hypotension was induced by nitroprusside.

Postoperatively, the patient did well and was discharged on June 1, after eight days without receiving medication. She was examined in the clinic on June 8 and on November 13, 1979, and was reported to be doing well on both visits.

Patient 2: an arteriovenous malformation (AVM)

The second patient first came to the Sloane Hospital on July 13, 1973, as a 14-year-old with a documented AVM in the right parietal area. Over the next few years, she was followed in the Neurology Clinic for headaches, stiff neck, and possible seizures. On July 19, 1974, she had a right parietal craniotomy, and feeders from the right cerebral artery were ligated.

Ten days later, she had a grand mal seizure. Because the procedure had not been totally successful, the patient continued to be followed in the Neurology Clinic. In May 1978, when she was hospitalized with a bleed from the AVM, pregnancy was diagnosed. A cerebral angiogram revealed the malformation was larger now, occupying the posterior aspect of the corpus callosum, with some extension into the choroid plexus of the third and lateral ventricles. She improved, and on June 14, 1978, had a D&C under local anesthesia for therapeutic abortion. The fetal age was approximately 10 weeks.

She was readmitted shortly after this procedure for possible corrective surgery of the AVM. When it was explained to her that there was a possibility of brain damage or death, and that the overall problem might still not be corrected, she refused the surgery and was discharged.

On April 13, 1979, in the Neurology Clinic, another pregnancy was diagnosed. The patient did not want therapeutic abortion. She was first seen in the Sloane Screening Clinic on May 15 with a 16-week-size uterus. On June 12, the patient probably had another small subarachnoid hemorrhage. But she did well, and continued to be followed in the Sloane Medical Clinic and in the Neurology Clinic. Her expected date of confinement was October 31, 1979. Her Pap smear was class I; rubella titer was 1:8; fasting and two-hour post-prandial blood sugars were normal; her hematocrit was 34.3%. Her serologic test for lues was negative; and SMA-6 and SMA-12 were normal.

On October 3, an ultrasound exam to determine fetal age displayed a biparietal diameter of 8.5 cm, consistent with 35 weeks. We were concerned about the effect of labor on her blood pressure, and the possibility that she might have subarachnoid hemorrhage from the AVM during labor. Also, she was found to be carrying a breech presentation. Therefore on October 21, we delivered a 3,080-gm male with Apgar scores of 8, 9, and 9 from the right sacrotransverse position by a low, flat, elliptical cesarean section, with a blood loss of approximately 1,000 ml.

The patient did well, and she was discharged on the sixth postoperative day. She was seen in the outpatient department on November 15 and December 3, 1979, when she was described as doing well. She was not put on birth control measures.

Neurologic problems of aneurysms and AVMs during pregnancy

ANTUNES: The clinical symptoms in both instances were typical of subarachnoid hemorrhage—headaches, vomiting, clouding of consciousness, and photophobia. But, as a rule, the diagnosis should be confirmed by lumbar puncture. Now, a CAT scan of the head is obtained as soon as possible, because blood in the intracranial cavity can be easily recognized.

The first patient had an area of increased density in the septal region and inside the third ventricle, thus confirming the presence of an intracranial hemorrhage [Figure 17-1]. Once such a diagnosis is made, it is mandatory

Figure 17-1.

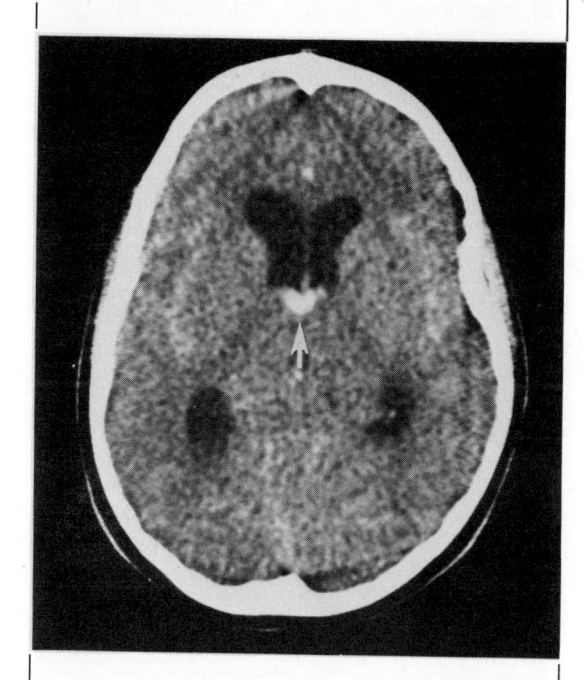

CAT scan of patient 1 confirms intracranial hemorrhage. Arrow points to area of increased density caused by the presence of blood within the third ventricle.

to find the source of the bleeding. Frequently, there is a ruptured intracranial aneurysm, and because these are multiple in about 20% of the cases, a complete angiographic study is necessary. This is now accomplished through the femoral route. In this patient, injection into the carotid arteries failed to demonstrate any abnormality, except some vasospasm. A vertebral injection, however, showed an aneurysm of the posterior-inferior cerebellar artery [Figure 17-2, upper].

There is another most unusual and interesting aspect to this angiogram. In later phases [Figure 17-2, lower], the angiographic dye has extravasated into the subarachnoid space—filling the fourth ventricle, the cisterna magna, and the subarachnoid space of the upper cervical region. This shows that the aneurysm ruptured again during angiography.

Dr. Finster asked me why I did not call the second patient's lesion an angioma. Well, AVMs are not tumors, but rather congenital maldevelopments made up of tortuous, enlarged arteries and veins, without an intermediary capillary network. There are direct shunts between feeding arteries and draining veins. Histologically, these vessels are dysplastic and do not show the normal layers.

Figure 17-2.

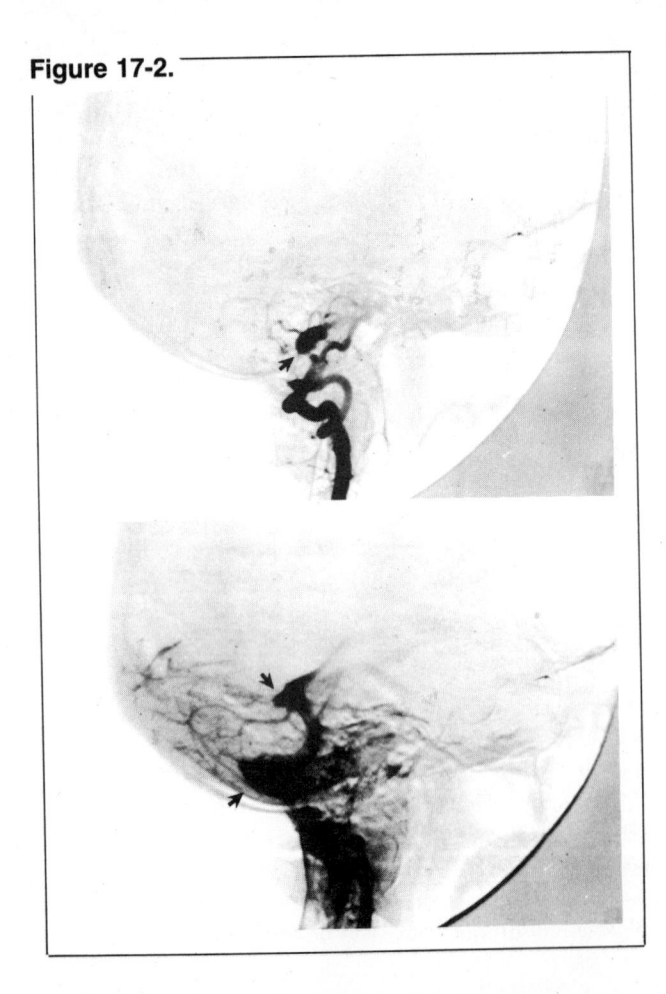

Sequence of cerebral angiograms shows rupture of aneurysm in patient 1. Upper: Dye from vertebral injection pinpoints source of bleeding (arrow) in posterior-inferior cerebellar artery. Lower: Rupture becomes apparent in later exposure. Dye has extravasated into cisterna magna (lower arrow) and fourth ventricle (upper arrow)

The patient with the AVM raised a most difficult question in terms of management. Her lesion was located in the thalamus, posterior corpus callosum, and roof of the third ventricle. As with intracranial aneurysms, to design a therapeutic plan, it is crucial to have a complete angiographic evaluation so one can trace the feeders, which commonly derive from multiple vessels. The AVM was being fed not only by branches of the anterior cerebral arteries, but also by branches of the posterior cerebral arteries—thalamo-perforating and posterior choroidal arteries—and drained into the internal cerebral vein and straight sinus [Figure 17-3].

When we saw this patient in 1974, we felt that a direct surgical attack on this lesion could possibly lead to a devastating neurologic deficit. We decided to occlude part of the lesion through embolization, a technique that

Drs. Sadek Hilal and W. Jost Michelsen have pioneered in our institute. The method consists of sending small Silastic or Gelfoam pellets (0.5 mm to 2 mm in diameter) into the feeding vessels, to take advantage of the particular hemodynamic conditions of these lesions. In this case, we were able to eliminate the major contributions from the posterior cerebral arteries. We then performed a craniotomy and clipped the major feeder from the anterior cerebral artery. A postoperative angiogram, however, showed a small residual AVM. Although we knew hemorrhage was still a risk, we did not think there was anything more we could do at that time.

Natural history of aneurysms and AVMs

Intracranial aneurysms typically appear in the arteries of the base that forms the circle of Willis. They are much more frequent in the anterior circulation, in the internal carotid artery and its branches, than in the distribution of the vertebro-basilar artery. Rarely do we see an aneurysm located posteriorly.

The initial mortality from a ruptured intracranial aneurysm is about 25%; of the survivors, 25% to 35% will bleed a second time, mostly during the following two weeks, and mortality

Figure 17-3.

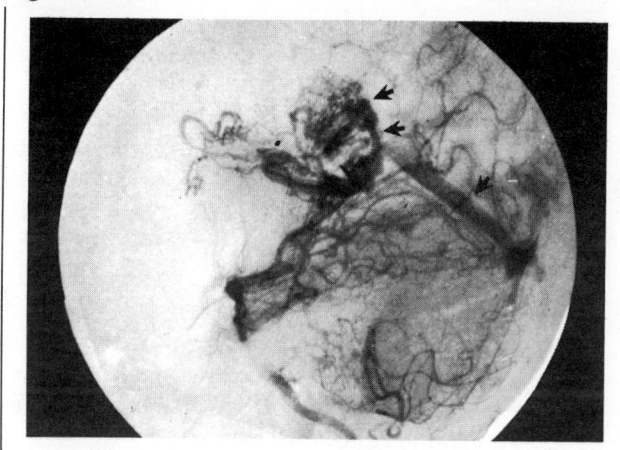

AVM in posterior thalamus of patient 2, fed by posterior choroidal arteries (upper two arrows), drains into straight sinus (lower arrow) as a result of shunt

from the second hemorrhage is around 20%. Because nothing can be done about the initial bleeding, we try to attack the aneurysm before the second bleeding occurs. Theoretically, surgery should be performed as soon as possible following the first bleeding. But we get best results when surgery is delayed (as with our first patient) until edema and vasospasm subside. In our institute, we wait until approximately the seventh or 10th day after hemorrhage.

We try to reduce the risks of another rupture by placing the patient in a quiet, darkened room; using appropriate sedatives and analgesics; and adding hypotensive, steroid, and anticonvulsant drugs. Recently, we have given antifibrinolytic agents such as aminocaproic acid to prevent lysis of the clot that plugs the hole in the aneurysm sac. When a patient with a ruptured intracranial aneurysm is pregnant, possible effects on mother and fetus will affect drug choice.

The first patient was particularly fortunate in surviving two bleeds, especially the one that occurred during angiography—a most unusual and, according to a recent review, most lethal event.[1] Why aneurysms rupture during angiography is unclear. Perhaps intraluminal or systemic blood pressures rise during the injection. Contrast medium of high osmolarity in the subarachnoid space seems to have a toxic effect on the neural tissue.

AVMs raise difficult problems. They may bleed repeatedly without causing a serious neurologic deficit, but there is always a cumulative risk, and the long-term prognosis is not always bright. Whenever possible, the treatment of choice for these lesions is surgery alone or preceded by embolization and, possibly, radiotherapy. All play a role.

Subarachnoid hemorrhages that occur during pregnancy do not, in clinical terms, differ from hemorrhages that happen in other situations. They are certainly not uncommon, occurring in about 1:2,000 to 1:7,000 pregnancies, and are responsible for 4.4% of maternal deaths. In a series reported by Amias, ruptured aneurysm was the cause of 21 deaths, AVM of 19, and other miscellaneous causes of 12.[2] That the proportion of ruptured AVMs is larger than in a comparable group of nonpregnant women suggests hemodynamic changes of pregnancy may play an important role.

The medical and neurosurgical management of these patients raises specific problems not only in the use of drugs. During the surgical procedures, we now routinely use controlled hypotension, hyperventilation, and diuretic agents such as mannitol.

Therapeutic dilemmas

FINSTER: I would like to comment on one aspect of subarachnoid hemorrhage occurring

Table 17-1. Time of occurrence of spontaneous intracranial hemorrhage in pregnancy*

| | Minn. Mat. Mortality Study | Number of cases reported | | | Totals |
		Pedowitz & Perell (review)	Copelan & Mabon	Amias	
During labor	3	1	1	0	5
Immediately postpartum	1 (1 hr)	2 ("immediate")	1 (3 hr)	3 (< 24 hr)	7
During pregnancy	16	26	3	40	85
> 24 hours postpartum	17	3	1	9	30
Totals	37	32	6	52	127

*Adapted from Freeman and Barno.[5]

during pregnancy: Frequently it is misdiagnosed as atypical toxemia. Raised intracranial pressure may cause convulsions and arterial hypertension; proteinuria may be due to irritation of the floor of the fourth ventricle. Indeed, our first patient was classified as toxemic because of elevated blood pressure and unexplained tachycardia.

As Dr. Antunes has already mentioned, the ratio of aneurysms to AVMs as causes of subarachnoid hemorrhage during pregnancy is approximately 50:50. The relatively low contribution of aneurysms can be explained by the fact that the incidence of bleeding from aneurysms increases with age, whereas pregnancy occurs most often in the third decade of life.

During gestation, the occurrence of subarachnoid hemorrhage seems to correlate with hemodynamic changes in the mother. Aneurysms tend to bleed most frequently during the third trimester in association with

141

peak increases in blood volume; hemorrhage from an AVM occurs most often during the second trimester, after the cardiac output and stroke volume have risen markedly.

We had to decide the order of procedures for the patient with the aneurysm. Craniotomy before delivery would have exposed the fetus to risks of the procedure, which also involves induction of hypotension. Even though there are reports in the literature indicating intact survival of the fetus following this type of surgery, in those few cases in which the fetal heart was monitored, maternal hypotension was associated with fetal bradycardia. Terminating the pregnancy before neurosurgical intervention, however, exposes the mother to the risk of another hemorrhage.

This point is well illustrated in Table 17-1. Of 127 spontaneous hemorrhages, five occurred during labor and seven within 24 hours of delivery. This information, more than any other, led us to deliver the patient by an elective cesarean section in the operating room of the Neurological Institute and carry out craniotomy immediately thereafter. Elective cesarean section allowed coordination of both surgical procedures, without the risk of labor's attendant increases in blood pressure and cardiac output. Most importantly, we avoided the perils of bearing-down efforts.

Figure 17-4 demonstrates changes in blood pressure and central venous pressure associated with the Valsalva maneuver. An increase in intrathoracic pressure leads to an increase in central venous and arterial pressures. As the venous return to the heart diminishes, however, the cardiac output and blood pressure begin to fall very rapidly. When bearing down ceases, there is a further decline in arterial pressure—because great vessels in the thorax are no longer compressed— and syncope may occur.

Finally, with unimpeded venous return, the cardiac output increases and so does the blood pressure. During the bearing-down effort, arterial as well as cerebrospinal fluid pressure increases.

As a result of this, there is no increase in the transmural pressure of the cerebral vasculature. This is no longer the case when the rise in blood pressure follows the cessation of the Valsalva maneuver, thus becoming critical as far as cerebral vascular abnormalities are concerned.

Our management of the patient with the aneurysm may seem to contradict recommenda-

Figure 17-4. Cardiovascular changes as mother bears down in second stage of labor*

Time (2-sec intervals)

Blood pressure (mm Hg)

Central venous pressure (mm Hg)

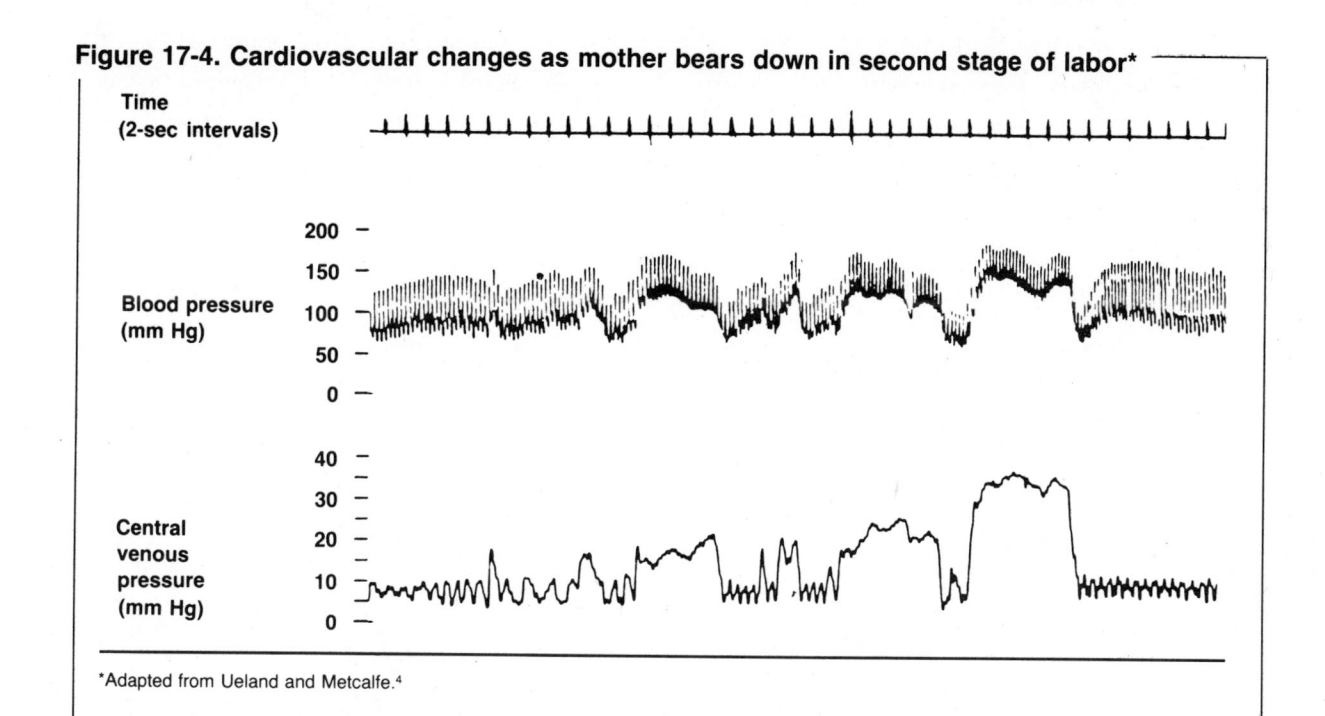

*Adapted from Ueland and Metcalfe.[4]

tions of many authors, including Pool, that neurosurgical correction should precede termination of pregnancy. I believe that their views can be modified when hemorrhage occurs after the 30th week of gestation. Today, we have means of determining (even inducing) fetal maturity and caring for the premature infant in the nursery. In our patient, the hemorrhage occurred during the 32nd week of gestation, and, by the time the neurosurgeons were ready to operate, the fetus was approximately 36 weeks old.

Dr. Petrie will discuss some of the obstetric problems and then I'll say a few words about the choice of anesthesia.

PETRIE: Figure 17-5 shows blood pressure changes that can occur during labor. This is a set of data on a rhesus monkey. Now, it's hard to get a monkey in labor to cooperate, but if she happened to begin pushing at the peak of a contraction, the arterial blood pressure could be raised quite a bit. This elevation could possibly bring about a bleed in the vascular system supplying the brain. Most obstetricians would agree that labor should be avoided in these situations.

Regarding the choice of performing the cesarean section or the craniotomy first, I agree with Dr. Finster's reasoning. Many of the fetuses may have to be delivered between the 28th and 36th week. To subject them to a hypotensive situation could induce hypoxia and certainly would not enhance pulmonary maturity should it be necessary to deliver them immediately.

A high CO_2 level with lowered O_2 level may lead to a state of respiratory distress. It is proper to take care of the fetus first when you can control blood pressure and potential hypoxia. Then, you can use procedures that may require hypotension for the craniotomy.

Choice of anesthesia

FINSTER: We used lumbar epidural anesthesia for both patients. During labor, regional anesthesia can buffer, to a degree, maternal hemodynamic changes—mainly by alleviating pain. Dr. Antunes mentioned the importance of controlling the blood pressure. This is difficult with light general anesthesia used for cesarean section.

For the neurosurgical procedure, this patient was very carefully anesthetized with morphine and large doses of sedative drugs before her trachea was intubated. Thus, the technique for preventing hypertension would definitely have depressed the newborn, had we applied it before delivery. Another important reason we chose regional anesthesia was that there is a sudden increase in the central vascular blood volume following delivery because of relieved pressure on the vena cava, contraction of the uterus, and expulsion of the placenta. The resulting increase can be avoided, or at least buffered, with the use of regional anesthesia simply because, with peripheral vasodilation and pooling, less blood is thrown into the central circulation. Indeed, for the patient with the AVM, epidural anesthesia was used not only for the cesarean section but also was continued in the recovery room for about 3 to 4 hours, to control blood pressure.

Comments and questions

VANDE WIELE: The claim has been made that because there is an increased frequency of rupture and bleeding as pregnancy progresses, one should consider cerebral aneurysm to be an indication for the interruption of pregnancy. Do you have any feeling on that?

ANTUNES: There continues to be a bit of a controversy about the timing of hemorrhage during pregnancy. Pool found a peak in aneurysm bleeding between 20 and 30 weeks.[3] Amias showed that hemorrhages from AVM were scattered throughout pregnancy, whereas aneurysms were more likely to rupture during the second half.[2] I believe, however, that more data are needed to clarify this question. The timing of surgery for an AVM is not as crucial as for a ruptured aneurysm, where the risk of recurrent bleeding is always present. The ideal surgical candidate is the patient without neurologic deficit (grade I), normal spinal fluid pressure, and no vasospasm in the angiogram. Surgical mortality in such patients is now around 2% to 3%.

FINSTER: Usually, it is recommended that the aneurysm be surgically attacked if the lesion is accessible. If the diagnosis is made during pregnancy, the patient will be operated on as soon as conditions allow it. Pregnancy should be terminated before craniotomy if the fetus is mature enough to have a good chance of survival. When a lesion is not accessible, there is no need to intervene or interrupt pregnancy.

ANTUNES: Timing of surgery for an AVM is not as important because the natural history is different. For aneurysms, timing becomes crucial. There's a high incidence of rebleeding, and that's what concerns us. The incidence of rebleeding increases by the seventh to the 14th day after the initial episode; by the fifth week after the initial hemorrhage, the incidence is lower. Then, there is a cumulative risk of about 5% per year. So timing becomes a statistical gamble, up to a certain point. If the patient is neurologically grade I, if the pressure of spinal fluid is normal, and if there is no vasospasm demonstrated by angiogra-

Figure 17-5. Correlation of arterial blood pressure and uterine contractions

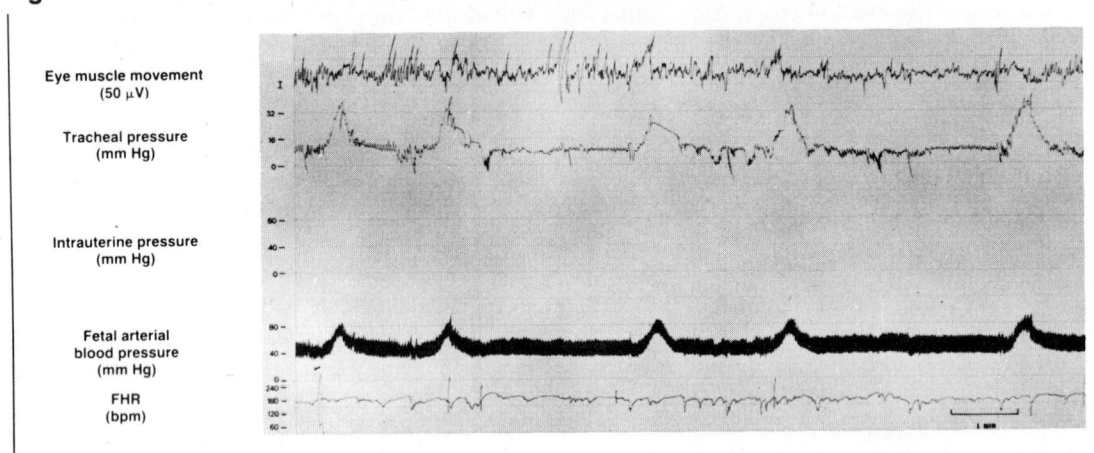

Eye muscle movement (50 μV)

Tracheal pressure (mm Hg)

Intrauterine pressure (mm Hg)

Fetal arterial blood pressure (mm Hg)

FHR (bpm)

Although there is no catheter in amniotic sac, tracheal and fetal arterial BP reflect intrauterine pressure (contractions). Catheter in arterial side of circulatory system demonstrates BP rises significantly during contractions. During labor, such elevation could bring about a subsequent bleed (rhesus monkey data)

phy, then she becomes an ideal candidate for surgery. Overall mortality for such patients is around 3%. So, surgery is a very acceptable thing. Agreed?

BARRON: Would you have counseled the patient with the AVM against becoming pregnant in the first place?

ANTUNES: Absolutely. Unfortunately, she is an immature young girl who has also refused any kind of contraceptive aids. The risk of rebleeding, of course, is still present and a repeat angiogram has shown the lesion has grown. Repeat embolization should be attempted, but the patient has refused it.

FENTON: Within the past six weeks, we had a patient with an aneurysm die. She came to North Shore University Hospital [Manhasset, N.Y.] with a bleed that occurred two weeks previously. She was about 34 weeks pregnant. After 36 hours, it became obvious that she was going downhill; hypertension and some proteinuria were present. We performed a cesarean section, but her condition deteriorated and she died about 10 days later. At the time of the section, she was almost brain dead.

ANTUNES: Well, the mortality in cases that we call grade IV (no spontaneous respirations, no brainstem reflexes) is close to 100%. There is no reason to intervene in such cases unless a large intracerebral hematoma is demonstrated. The CAT scan is now indispensable for such diagnosis. Evacuation of the blood clot and clipping of the aneurysm, if accessible, have occasionally been successful, but the prognosis is generally hopeless.

FINSTER: A team approach including the obstetrician, neurosurgeon, anesthesiologist, and neonatologist is absolutely essential. The happy outcome of both patients we have discussed today illustrates it particularly well. Thank you very much.

REFERENCES
1. Koenig GH, Marshall WH Jr, Poole GJ, et al: Rupture of intracranial aneurysms during cerebral angiography: report of ten cases and review of the literature. Neurosurgery 5:314, 1979
2. Amias AG: Cerebral vascular disease in pregnancy. I. Haemorrhage. J Obstet Gynaecol Br Commonw 77:100, 1970
3. Pool JL: Treatment of intracranial aneurysms during pregnancy. JAMA 192:209, 1965
4. Ueland K, Metcalfe J: Circulatory changes in pregnancy. Clin Obstet Gynecol 18:41, 1975
5. Freeman DW, Barno A: Letter: Berry aneurysms. Obstet Gynecol 45:601, 1975

Index

A

Abdominal problems, management, 37-47
  adhesions, 42
  appendicitis, 37-39
  cholecystitis, 43-44
  gallbladder disease, 43-44
  gallstones, 43-44
  intestinal obstruction, 41-43
  intussusception, 43
  ovarian cysts, 39-40
  pancreatitis, 45-47
  peptic ulcer disease, 44-45
  salpingitis, 40-41
  tubo-ovarian abscess, 40-41
  volvulus, midgut, 43
Abortion,
  acute renal failure and, 10, 11
  septic, 10, 11
Abruptio placentae
  acute renal failure and, 10, 11
  eclampsia and, 101
Abscesses
  pelvic: *see* Pelvic abscesses
  tubo-ovarian, 40-41
Acute renal failure: *see* Renal failure, acute
Adhesions, intestinal obstruction and, 42
Adnexectomy, bilateral, for ruptured pelvic abscess, 77
Allergic reactions to anesthetics, 6, 25-26
Amniocentesis, in eclampsia, 104
Amniotic fluid embolism
  acute renal failure and, 10, 11
  cardiorespiratory complications, 35
Amniotomy, eclamptic patient, 104
Anemia, microangiopathic hemolytic, postpartum renal failure and, 10, 11
Anovulatory bleeding: *see* Bleeding, anovulatory
Anesthesia
  paracervical block, prolonged fetal bradycardia and, 96
  for subarachnoid hemorrhage, 144-145
  total spinal, emergencies in, 23-25
Anesthesiology, emergency training for ob/gyn residents, 50
Anesthetic emergencies, 17-26
  airway control, 17-21
  laryngoscopy, 18-21
  local anesthetics, reactions, 25-26
  obesity, 17-18
  pulmonary aspiration, 21-23
  regurgitation, 21-23
  total spinal anesthesia, 23-25
  tracheal intubation, 18-21
Anesthetics, local
  allergic reactions, 25-26
  recommended dosage, 24-25
  toxic and allergic reactions, 25-26
Anesthetic toxicity, vasovagal syncope and, 6
Antimicrobial therapy: *see* specific infectious condition
Apgar scoring system, for distressed newborn, 118

149

Appendicitis, 37-39
Arteriovenous malformations, 135-147
   see also Hemorrhage, subarachnoid
Asphyxia: see Distressed newborn
Aspiration, meconium, distressed newborn, 121
Aspiration, pulmonary
   acid, 22
   anesthetic emergencies, 21-23
   food particles, 22
   infection and, 23
   therapy and management, 23
Aspiration pneumonitis, 33-34

B

Bacterial endocarditis, acute renal failure and, 11
Biopsy, vaginal hemorrhage and, 80, 83
Birth control medication: see Contraceptives, oral
Bleeding: see Bleeding, anovulatory; see also Hemorrhage; Shock, hemorrhagic
Bleeding, anovulatory, 85-90
   abnormal bleeding patterns, 86
   D&C, 87, 89
   definition of problem, 85-87
   dysfunctional uterine, 85-87
   endometrial, 85
   estrogen breakthrough, 86-87
   estrogen-progesterone withdrawal-bleeding response, 85-90
   estrogen therapy, 90
   hysterosalpingography, 90
   hysteroscopy, 90
   medical management, 85-90
   oral contraceptives, therapeutic use, 87-90
   progestational breakthrough, 86-87
   progestational therapy, 87-90
   progestational withdrawal bleeding, 89
   progestin-estrogen oral contraceptives, therapeutic use, 87-89
   progestin therapy, 90
   recurrent, 90
   spontaneous ovulation, 88
   therapy, choice of, 87-90
Blood replacement therapy, for coagulation failure, 59
Bradycardia, fetal: see Fetal bradycardia
Brain, complications associated with eclampsia, 101
Bronchoscopy, indications for, in pulmonary aspiration, 22

C

Cardiac massage, closed-chest, for distressed newborn, 119
Cardiopulmonary resuscitation: see Resuscitation
Cardiorespiratory complications, 27-35
   adult cardiorespiratory distress syndrome, 30, 33-35
   arrhythmias, 31-32
   atrial fibrillation, 33
   bradycardia, fetal: see Fetal bradycardia
   changes in cardiorespiratory system, 27-28
   heart problems, 28-33
   ischemic events, characteristic ECG forms, 32
   lung involvement, 33-35
   management, 27-35
   molar pregnancy syndrome, postevacuation, 34-35
   myocardial infarction, acute, 31
   myocardial ischemia, 31-32
   neonatal: see Distressed newborn
   pulmonary aspiration: see Aspiration, pulmonary
   pulmonary edema, acute, 28-30
   pulmonary embolus, 34
   reversal of intracardiac shunt, 30-31
   rheumatic heart disease, 33
   ventricular ectopic beats, 30, 32

Cardiovascular changes
  in second stage of labor, 143
  subarachnoid hemorrhage and, 143
Cardiovascular collapse, in newborn, 120-121
Cardiovascular depression, anesthesia-induced, 25
Central nervous system
  alterations, in eclampsia, 101
  depression, anesthesia-induced, 25
Cerebral aneurysm, 133-147
  see also Hemorrhage, subarachnoid
Cerebral edema, eclampsia and, 101
Cerebral hemorrhage, eclampsia and, 101
Cerebrovascular accident, eclampsia and, 101
Cesarean section
  eclamptic patient, 104-105
  uterine rupture, 111-112
Cholecystitis, acute, 43-44
Chorioamnionitis, acute renal failure and, 10, 11
Choriocarcinoma, vaginal hemorrhage and, 79-80, 83
Coagulation, disseminated intravascular
  acute renal failure and, 10, 11
  eclampsia and, 101
Coagulation defects, acute renal failure and, 10, 11
Coagulation failure, blood replacement therapy, in hemorrhagic shock, 59
Colonic tumor, vaginal hemorrhage and, 90
Contraceptive devices, intrauterine, as cause of ectopic pregnancy, 64-65
Contraceptives, oral
  for control of anovulatory bleeding, 87-90
  ectopic pregnancy and, 65-66
  gallstones and, 43
Convulsions: see Seizures
Cricothyrotomy, in anesthetic emergencies, 21
Culdocentesis
  ectopic pregnancy, 68
  ruptured pelvic abscesses, 74-75
Cysts, ovarian, 39-40

D

D & C
  anovulatory bleeding, 87, 89
  ectopic pregnancy, 68
  endometrial hemorrhage, 81-82
  leukemia, acute, 83, 84
Diethylstilbestrol, vaginal bleeding and, 79

Distressed newborn
  Apgar scoring system, 118
  asphyxia, 115-121
  bradycardia, fetal: see Fetal bradycardia
  cardiovascular collapse, 120-121
  closed-chest cardiac massage, 119
  counseling, maternal, 122
  fast action for, 115-123
  hydrops fetalis, 121-122
  meconium aspiration, 121
  metabolic acidosis, 119
  neurovascular response, 120
  resuscitation techniques and equipment, 115-120, 122
  shock, 120-121

E

Eclampsia, 99-105
  acute hypertension and, 100-101
  amniocentesis, 104
  amniotomy, 104
  antihypertensive drugs, 103
  central nervous system alterations, 101
  cerebral hemorrhage, 101
  complications, 101
  control, strategies for, 99-105
  delivery, rules for, 103-105

151

diagnosis, 101
glomeruloendotheliosis and, 100
magnesium sulfate therapy, 99, 102-104
mortality, maternal and fetal, 99, 101
pathophysiology, 100-101
preeclampsia and, 100, 101
preeclampsia-eclampsia, acute renal failure and, 10, 11
premature fetus, delivery, 104-105
renal function, 100-101
seizures, 101, 103
toxemia, eclamptogenic, hemorrhagic shock and, 56
treatment, 101-104
Ectopic pregnancy, 63-69
causes, 65-66
culdocentesis, 68
D & C, 68
detection and diagnosis, 63-69
fallopian tube, partial occlusion, 64
fallopian tube surgery, effects, 66
incidence, 63-65
intrauterine devices and, 64-65
laparoscopy, 68
mortality, 63
pain, location and frequency, 66-67
pregnancy testing, 66
radioimmunoassay, 66
radioreceptor assay, 66
salpingectomy, 68
salpingostomy, 69
sites, 64-65
surgical approaches, 68-69
treatment, 63-69
ultrasound, diagnostic, 66
Edema: *see* Cerebral edema; Pulmonary edema
Embolus
amniotic fluid, 35
pulmonary, 34
Emergency training for ob/gyn residents, 49-54
anesthesiology, 50
recommended programs, 52-54
specialization, 50-52
Endocarditis, bacterial, 11
Endometrial bleeding: *see* Bleeding, anovulatory; Hemorrhage, vaginal
Endometrial tumor, vaginal hemorrhage and, 80
Endometritis, postpartum, 125-131
antimicrobial therapy, 128-130
causative organisms, 126-127
cultures, 127-128
diagnosis, 127
differential diagnosis, 127
epidemiology, 130-131
incidence, 125
predisposing factors, 125-126

Estrogen: *see also* Contraceptives, oral
therapy, for anovulatory bleeding, 87-90
Estrogen breakthrough bleeding, 86-87
Estrogen-progesterone withdrawal-bleeding response, 85-90
Exenteration, vaginal hemorrhage following, 82-83

F

Fallopian tube
partial occlusion, ectopic pregnancy and, 64
surgery, ectopic pregnancy and, 66
Fertility potential, after surgery for ruptured pelvic abscess, 77
Fetal asphyxia: *see* Distressed newborn
Fetal bradycardia, 91-97
assessment by fetal heart rate, 94-96
assessment by scalp blood sampling, 93-96
basic guidelines, 91-93
heart block and, 96
heart rate decelerations, classification. 92-93
heart rate variability, 91-97
hypoxia and, 91

management, 93-97
prolonged, following paracervical block anesthesia, 96
Fetal death: see Mortality, fetal
Fetal distress: see Distressed newborn
Fetal hydrops: 121-122
Fever, postpartum, 126-127

G

Gallbladder disease, 43-44
Gallstones, 43-44
    pancreatitis and, 46
Glomeruloendotheliosis, eclampsia and, 100, 101
Glomerulonephritis, acute renal failure and, 11

H

Heart problems: see Cardiorespiratory complications
Heart rate, fetal: see Fetal bradycardia
Hemolysis, in acute renal failure, 10, 11
Hemorrhage: see also Bleeding; Shock, hemorrhagic
    acute renal failure and, 10, 11
    definition, 79
    postpartum, 10, 11
Hemorrhage, cerebral, eclampsia and, 101
Hemorrhage, subarachnoid, 133-147

anesthesia, choice of, 144-145
arteriovenous malformation, 135-147
cardiovascular changes in second stage of labor, 143
cerebral aneurysm, 133-147
correlation of arterial blood pressure and uterine contractions, 146
counseling, for avoidance of pregnancy, 146
mortality, 147
natural history, 139-140
neurologic problems, 136-139
spontaneous, time of occurrence, 141
surgery, timing of, 145
termination of pregnancy, 145
therapeutic dilemmas, 140-144
timing of, during pregnancy, 145
Hemorrhage, vaginal, 79-84
    associated conditions, 79-80
    cancer, 79-80
    choriocarcinoma, 83
    coping with, 79-84
    D & C, 81-82
    diethylstilbestrol and, 79
    endometrial, control, 81-82
    hypogastric ligation, 80-81
    irradiation, 80-81
    leukemia, acute, 83, 84
    molar pregnancy, 81

    platelet count, 83
    postbiopsy, 80, 83
    postexenteration, 82-83
    postoperative, 80
    prevention, 83
    risk of, 79-80
    solid tumors, 84
    uterine, 80
Hydrops fetalis, 121-122
Hyperemesis gravidarum, 10, 11
Hypertension
    acute, eclampsia and, 100-101
    acute renal failure and, 9
Hyperventilation, and vasovagal syncope, differential diagnosis, 6
Hypofibrinogenemia, eclampsia and, 101
Hypogastric arteries, ligation
    for cervical and vaginal hemorrhage, 80-81
    for hemorrhagic shock, 61
Hysterectomy
    pelvic abscess, ruptured, 77
    uterine rupture, 112-113
    vaginal hemorrhage, postoperative, 80
Hysterosalpingography, for diagnosis of recurrent anovulatory bleeding, 90
Hysteroscopy, for diagnosis of anovulatory bleeding, 90
Hysterotomy, for uterine rupture, 111

I

Infection: *see also* Sepsis
  endometritis, postpartum, 125-131
Intestinal obstruction, acute, 41-43
Intracardiac shunt, reversal of, 30-31
Intubation, tracheal, in anesthetic emergencies, 18-21
Intussusception, intestinal, 43
Ischemia
  acute renal failure and, 10, 11
  characteristic ECG forms, 32
  myocardial: *see* Myocardial ischemia
IUDs: *see* Contraceptive devices, intrauterine

L

Laparoscopy, for ectopic pregnancy, 68
Laparotomy, for ruptured pelvic abscess, 76
Laryngoscopy, in anesthetic emergencies, 18-21
Leukemia, acute, vaginal hemorrhage and, 83, 84
Liver
  complications associated with eclampsia, 101
  fatty, acute renal failure and, 10, 11

Lungs: *see* Cardiorespiratory complications

M

Magnesium sulfate therapy, for eclampsia, 99, 102-104
Meconium aspiration, distressed newborn, 121
Metabolic acidosis, distressed newborn, 119
Molar pregnancy
  postevacuation, cardiorespiratory complications, 34-35
  vaginal hemorrhage and, 81
Mortality, fetal
  eclampsia, 99, 101
  renal failure, maternal, 10, 11
  uterine rupture, 113
Mortality, maternal
  acute renal failure, 11-12
  eclampsia, 99, 101
  ectopic pregnancy, 63
  hemorrhagic shock, 55, 56
  pelvic abscess, ruptured, 72
  subarachnoid hemorrhage, 147
  uterine rupture, 111, 113
Myocardial infarction, vasovagal syncope and, 6-7
Myocardial ischemia, cardiorespiratory complications, 31-32

N

Necrosis
  acute tubular, renal failure and, 11
  bilateral cortical, acute and chronic renal failure, 10-12
  periportal, eclampsia and, 101
Neurologic problems, subarachnoid hemorrhage and, 136-139
Neurovascular response, neonatal, to asphyxia, 120
Newborn, distressed: *see* Distressed newborn

O

Obesity, airway control problems, 17-18
Ob/gyn training: *see* Emergency training for ob/gyn residents
Oral contraceptives: *see* Contraceptives, oral
Ovarian cysts, 39-40
Ovarian tumor, 80
Ovulation, spontaneous, in anovulatory patient, 88

P

Pancreatitis
  acute, 45-47
  necrotizing or hemorrhagic type, 47

Pelvic abscesses, ruptured, 71-77
   aids in diagnosis and management, 74-75
   antimicrobial therapy, 75
   culdocentesis, 74-75
   differential diagnosis, 73
   fertility potential, postoperative, 77
   laparotomy, 76
   medical management, 75-76
   mortality rate, 72
   peritonitis and, 72-77
   risks of, and incidence, 71-72
   serum chemistries and enzymes, 74
   signs and symptoms, 72-73
   sonography, 74
   surgery, 71-77
   urinalysis, 74
   x-rays, 74
Peptic ulcer disease, 44-45
   perforations, symptoms, stages of, 45
   peritonitis, 45
Peritonitis
   pelvic abscesses, ruptured, 72-77
   peptic ulcer, perforated, 45
Placenta previa, acute renal failure and, 10, 11
Platelet count, and vaginal hemorrhage, relationship, 83-84
Pneumonitis, aspiration, 33-34
Postpartum endometritis: *see* Endometritis, postpartum
Preeclampsia-eclampsia: *see* Eclampsia
Pregnancy testing, for ectopic pregnancy, 66
Progestational breakthrough bleeding, 86
Progestational therapy
   for anovulatory bleeding, 90
   postmenopausal, 87
Progestational withdrawal bleeding, for anovulatory bleeding, 89
Progesterone oral contraceptives: *see* Contraceptives, oral
Progestin-estrogen oral contraceptives: *see* Contraceptives, oral
Progestin therapy, for anovulatory bleeding, 90
Prostaglandins, for postpartum hemorrhage, 59
Pulmonary aspiration: *see* Aspiration, pulmonary
Pulmonary edema, acute, causes and management, 28-30
Pulmonary embolus, 34
Pulmonary problems, *see* Cardiorespiratory complications
Pyelonephritis
   acute renal failure and, 10, 11
   and appendicitis, differentiation, 39

R

Radioimmunoassay, for ectopic pregnancy, 66
Radioreceptor assay, for ectopic pregnancy, 66
Radiotherapy, for cervical and vaginal hemorrhage, 80-81
Regurgitation, anesthetic emergency, 21-23
Renal complications associated with eclampsia, 100-101
Renal failure, acute, 9-15
   associated conditions, 10-12
   diagnosis of specific syndrome, 10-12
   dialysis, hemo- or peritoneal, criteria for choosing, 13-14
   fetal death, 11
   fluid status, clinical parameters, 13
   hypertension and, 9
   management, 9-15
   in nonpregnant state, causes, 11
   postpartum, 10-11
   pregnancy-associated conditions, 10-12
   prerenal and parenchymal renal disease, differentiation and management, 12
   therapeutic measures, 12-15
Renal failure, chronic, 11
Residents, ob/gyn, training: *see* Emergency training for ob/

gyn residents
Respiratory distress: *see* Cardiorespiratory complications; Distressed newborn
Resuscitation
  cardiopulmonary, for vasovagal syncope, 1-7
  distressed newborn, 115-120, 122
Rheumatic heart disease, 33

S

Salpingectomy, for ectopic pregnancy, 68
Salpingitis, 40-41
  and appendicitis, differentiation, 39
Salpingo-oophorectomy, for ruptured pelvic abscess, 76
Salpingostomy, for ectopic pregnancy, 69
Sarcoma botryoides, vaginal hemorrhage and, in children, 79
Seizures
  anesthesia-induced, 25-26
  eclamptic, 101, 103
Sepsis: *see also* Infection
  acute renal failure, 10, 11
  hemorrhagic shock, 56
  intra-abdominal, associated with ruptured pelvic abscesses, 75

puerperal, acute renal failure and, 10, 11
puerperal, streptococcal, 130-131
Sepsis-endotoxemia, acute renal failure and, 10, 11
Shock
  distressed newborn, 120-121
  perforated peptic ulcer, 45
Shock, hemorrhagic, 55-61
  see also Hemorrhage
  blood replacement therapy for coagulation failure, 59
  clinical picture, 56-57
  combating, general plan of action, 57-61
  eclamptogenic toxemia, 56
  evolution, 56-57
  hypogastric ligation, 61
  infusion, 58
  medical management, 58, 60
  monitoring patient, 58
  mortality, causes and incidence, 55, 56
  pathophysiology, 55-56
  postpartum, 58-59
  prostaglandin therapy, 59
  sepsis, 56
  surgical management, 58, 60-61
  transfusion therapy, 59-60
  treatment priorities, 55-61
  ventilation, 57-58
  volume challenge, 57

volume replacement, 57
Sonography: *see* Ultrasound, diagnostic
Subarachnoid hemorrhage: *see* Hemorrhage, subarachnoid

T

Toxemia, eclamptogenic, 56
Toxicity, anesthetic, 6, 25-26
Toxins, abortion, acute renal failure and, 10, 11
Training: *see* Emergency training for ob/gyn residents
Transfusion therapy, for hemorrhagic shock, 59-60
Tubo-ovarian abscess, 40-41
Tumors
  endometrial, 80
  ovarian, 80
  solid, 84

U

Ultrasound, diagnostic
  ectopic pregnancy, 66
  ruptured pelvic abscesses, 74
Urolithiasis, differential diagnosis, 39
Uterine bleeding: *see* Bleeding, anovulatory; Hemorrhage, vaginal
Uterine ruptures, 107-113
  causes, 109
  cesarean section, 111-112

classifications, 109
diagnosis, 110-111
hysterectomy, 112-113
hysterotomy, 111
incidence, 107-108
management, 111-113
mortality, fetal, 113
mortality, maternal, 111, 113
obstetric factors, 109
scarred type, 109-111
spontaneous type, 109, 111
traumatic type, 109, 111

V

Vaginal hemorrhage: *see* Hemorrhage, vaginal
Vasovagal syncope, 1-7
  airway establishment, 4
  anesthetic toxicity and, 6
  artificial circulation, production of, 5
  assessment, 4
  breathing, initiation of, 4-5
  cardiopulmonary resuscitation, 1-7
  differential diagnosis, 6-7
  drugs, 5
  electrical defibrillation, 7-8
  management, 4-6
  pathophysiology, 1-4
  prevention, guidelines, 7
  symptoms, 3
Ventricular ectopic beats, 30, 32
Volvulus, midgut, 43

Other Titles of Related Interest From Medical Economics Books

Management of High-Risk Pregnancy
John T. Queenan, M.D., Editor
ISBN 0-87489-221-X

Psychological Aspects of Gynecology and Obstetrics
Benjamin B. Wolman, Ph.D., Editor
ISBN 0-87489-009-8

Rape: Helping the Victim
Susan Halpern
ISBN 0-87489-010-1

Drugs Used With Neonates and During Pregnancy
Avrin M. Overbach, M.D., and Morton J. Rodman, Ph.D.
ISBN 0-87489-061-6

Human Disease in Color
Chandler Smith, M.D.
ISBN 0-87489-188-4

Ethical Options in Medicine
Gregory E. Pence, Ph.D.
ISBN 0-87489-233-3

Advances in Gynaecological Endocrinology
Royal College of Obstetricians and Gynaecologists
ISBN 0-87489-225-2

Diagnosis and Management of Neural Tube Defects
Royal College of Obstetricians and Gynaecologists
ISBN 0-87489-229-5

For information, write to:

Medical Economics Books
680 Kinderkamack Road
Oradell, New Jersey 07649